Raise
the
Barre

Introducing

CARDIO BARRE–

The Revolutionary 8-Week Program

for Total Mind/Body Transformation

Raise
the
Barre

Richard Giorla

with Laurel House

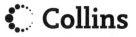
Collins
An Imprint of HarperCollinsPublishers

This book is written as a source of information only. The information contained in this book should by no means be considered a substitute for the advice of a qualified medical professional, who should always be consulted before beginning any new diet, exercise, or health program.

HarperCollins books may be purchased for educational, business, or sales promotional use. For information please write: Special Markets Department, HarperCollins Publishers, 10 East 53rd Street, New York, NY 10022.

FIRST EDITION

Designed by Jaime Putorti

Printed on acid-free paper

Library of Congress Cataloging-in-Publication Data has been applied for.

ISBN-10: 0-06-078662-0
ISBN-13: 978-0-06-078662-5

03 04 05 06 07 QW/WBC 10 9 8 7 6 5 4 3 2 1

Contents

Acknowledgments

There are just too many people to name who have contributed to the success of *Cardio Barre*. I give all of my thanks to my family, friends, clients, business associates, and everyone who gave their love, support, and wisdom to make all of this possible and make me strong. I would also like to thank those who gave no support or had little faith in me, for making me stronger. This is just to say that throughout life there will always be obstacles, challenges, and adversity . . . and anything is possible . . . dreams do come true. Follow your dreams!

My heartfelt thanks and love to the people who helped put this book together. Thank you to my editor, Sarah Durand, my agent, Michael Broussard, and Laurel House, who helped translate my passion into words.

Introduction

> *Life is not measured by the number of*
> *breaths you take, but by the number of*
> *moments that take your breath away.*
>
> —ANONYMOUS

Take a bow, Tae Bo; stop your wheels, Spinning; step aside, Pilates—there is a new fitness phenomenon in town. Cardio Barre is not just the fitness flavor-of-the-month, but rather a cutting-edge, body-burning, stretching and strengthening system that will change the way you view working out, while shaping you into your image of bodily perfection.

What you hold in your hands is the "hottest, new" in exercise. Cardio Barre has become the buzzword on the tips of trendsetter's tongues. Having consumed yoga, Pilates, Spinning, and Tae Bo long ago, exercise enthusiasts are now in need of something new to sink their teeth into. Celebrity trainers have tried to satisfy your exercise appetites, but their tips often turn out to be little more than old material made to look new. In an attempt to fill the fitness void, a profusion of diet books have filled our bookshelves, asking us to eliminate entire food groups. Whatever happened to balance? If you want a better body, you have to raise the bar, paying equal attention to healthy diet and exercise habits. Cardio Barre is new and unique and most important—effective. It will raise the bar in fitness, setting a new standard that all other fads will follow. This book is not about Band-Aid fixes or short cuts, it is about real, quickly achieved, long-lasting effects. I will provide the tools—the body basics, exercise techniques, and nutritional consultation—and illuminate the path to inspiration.

Give me 8 weeks and watch as your perfect body takes shape. The one thing in this world that you can control is yourself and your body. Take control right now. I will teach you how.

My name is Richard Giorla and I am the founder of Cardio Barre.

If you are reading this book, chances are that you are ready to make, or are at least thinking about, some sort of change in your life. You don't necessarily need to be struggling with weight issues to get something out of this. In fact, many of my students are lean. While I definitely work with women who are overweight, I also work with women and men who are trying to maintain their weight, tone up, or work on self-esteem. So whoever you are, whatever your issues may be, I am ready to take you on, if you are ready to make the commitment. The fact is that everyone struggles at one point in his or her life. I did. And everyone can also overcome the difficulties, leap over the hurdles, take steps to overcome defeat and actually be better because of it. Believe me, I know not only from the endless stories that I hear from my students, but also from personal experience. Yes, I too had to raise my own bar and crawl out of a potentially disastrous downward spiral that seemed to be swallowing up my energy, body, and enthusiasm to live the life I had always envisioned for myself.

Who Am I to Tell You . . . ?

I have always had a passion for dance, which can be difficult for a man. Not only is there typically little money in dance, but my father didn't exactly embrace it, nor did my "manly men" friends. Still, I persisted to pave my own path. I started out as a junior Olympic gymnast in Philadelphia. But my desire to dance on stage drove me to New York City to further my studies as a technical dancer. I dabbled in many forms of dance, from classical ballet and jazz to hip-hop and break dancing; I must admit, I even danced with the controversial group "Chippendales." In order to strengthen my arms and maintain my masculine physique, I learned from the body builders how to incorporate weight training into my regular workout routine.

In search of the intangible "something more," I took my talent to Los Angeles and was quickly embraced by the city notorious for fifteen minutes of fame. I had several stints as a professional dancer on stage, in films, on television shows, in commercials, and was hit by an unexpected yet always dreaded blow: I had been dancing with Michael Jackson, and other entertainment elite, and then performing in a show at Universal Studios, and eventually I pulled a groin muscle so severely that I was completely unable to dance for two years. This rigorous routine and my athleticism took a toll on my body—and the injury instantly ended my professional dancing career, stripping me of not only my livelihood but also my emotional lifeline.

Living off of credit cards, debt began to pile on top of me. Out of work and with an inability to exercise, my body began to lose its definition. Thanks to low-self esteem, financial stress, and lack of motivation to move my body at all, emotional pounds became physical pounds. I watched in disbelief as inches latched on to my body, leaching me of any remaining crumbs of confidence. With $80,000 hanging over my head from creditors and an unfamiliar body that was suddenly mine, I hopelessly wondered why my fifteen minutes had so suddenly come to an end. Los Angeles is a very sad and lonely city when luck is no longer on your side.

After months of listlessly retreating into an unhealthy shell, I realized that sitting around and doing nothing would do nothing for me. In order for my life to change, *I* had to change. I began simply by reopening my eyes and ears, ready to embrace any opportunity that might help me create a better life for myself. Unfortunately, no gifts from God presented themselves; but instead of wallowing away as a disenchanted ex-dancer, I knew that in order to take the next step, and in turn, take my life back, I first needed to heal. I went into a physical therapy program and began to study Pilates. After a few sessions, I began to regain my physical and mental strength enough to look for work. I was able to utilize my fitness knowledge and experience and turn it into a business. In an attempt to create the most perfect and thorough form of fitness, I took bits and pieces from my vast dance, exercise, and life knowledge and combined them into one comprehensive dance-based fitness program.

Cardio Barre utilizes the best elements of ballet, weight training, Pilates, yoga, and core work. With a program that was guaranteed to work, I opened my first Cardio Barre studio in Los Angeles in 2001. Quickly, my intimate studio was flooded with students—celebrities and stay-at-home moms alike—who swore that Cardio Barre was changing their lives. With a wait list for classes, I decided to expand rather than turn anyone away.

In a short period of time, my face was suddenly brandished throughout the pages of fitness, gossip, and celebrity magazines. Before I knew it, my success had turned into an empire, and I exuded confidence, strength, poise and passion, all in a matter of months.

What is so amazing is that I am a normal guy, an average Joe. Yet this average Joe was able to overcome what I had thought to be impassable obstacles and create something out of nothing. So can you. I am not saying it was an easy feat. But would I do it all again? Absolutely! Life is a never-ending journey. Enjoy every second of it. You may, at this moment, feel quite satisfied with who you are today. But there is always room for improvement. Why settle for less when you can have more?

Raise your bar. I did.

Life is not about finding yourself.
Life is about creating yourself.
—ANONYMOUS

Now, I promise you, Cardio Barre is not yet another fitness fad or passing exercise phenomenon guaranteeing empty results and broken promises. It is the newest, most effective and efficient way to work every inch of your body. Cardio Barre will not just change your body; it will seep into each and every crevice of your life, improving your attitude, relationships, habits, diet, mental state, sleep, emotional well-being, and day-to-day experience. Scientific studies and medicine prove that exercise is good for you. *Raise the Barre* will back up the statistics about cardio exercise, resistance training, healthful eating, and how they collaboratively make for a healthy you.

Cardio Barre can change your life, but only if you are truly ready for change. If you want to see proof, turn on the TV, or go to a movie or concert. Many of those flawless bodies covered in sexy curves and ripped with muscle definition, their presence forcing heads to turn each time they enter a room, those are my creations. You can be too.

Those healthy bodies are not created from exercise alone. Fifty percent of their perfection can be attributed to diet. *Raise the Barre* will teach you how to make wholesome food choices, without restricting entire food groups or completely ignoring unrelenting hankerings for a few of your favorite things. But the simple fact is that it takes approximately 3 weeks to break a habit. In those weeks, a bad habit can be discarded and a healthy one instilled. If chocolate is your unhealthy habit, after 3 weeks without it, you won't want it anymore. We will get into the nitty-gritty, but what you need to know now is that calories are the same for everyone, independent of your fitness level or athletic ability. If you are burning more calories than you are taking in, you are losing weight. With calories you cannot cheat, you cannot slack off. The harder you work, the more calories you burn, the more fat you lose. It is that simple!

*   *   *

If you think dancers and celebrities are born perfect, you are wrong. Rarely is a perfect body born; they are sculpted. I will guide you along the celebrity-laden path, teaching you the basics of muscular structure, instructing you on proper exercise methods, and giving enough techniques to help you to avoid injury. Be prepared to feel a little discomfort. You will be sore in the morning. And believe me, that is a good thing! You will work your body beyond your preconceived limitations. Your muscles may feel like they are ripping. You may cry out in frustration and in fear of self-defeat. You will get to your breaking point and you will consider sabotaging it all for fear of failure, or is it fear of success? You may need to take a hot bath just to get to sleep at night, and your muscles will scream at you in the morning as you jump up and do a few leg lifts before breakfast. Though you will undoubtedly suffer from pain, frustration, and multiple loads of sweat-soaked laundry, I guarantee that you will thank me once pounds and inches start dropping off your body and you are exuding confidence from each and every one of your pores.

Stars—be it celebrities, politicians, homecoming kings and queens, or dancing divas—at one point in their lives made the conscious choice to have that striking presence that fills a room when they enter it. They demand respect and attention, and they won't have it any other way. They decided it was their turn to raise their bar; and look how high they were able to push it. Now it's your turn. But the motivation and the drive must come from within you. I will teach you how to find and develop that inner inspiration, and eventually I will ask you to reach outside the book and within yourself, where you will find the trainer inside of you. Once your inner instructor emerges, you will learn to trust your instincts and listen to your body. You will have the sensitivity to hear the roar of your muscles when they beg for you to stop, or the whisper of your blood encouraging a faster flow. Yet you will simultaneously have the strength to conquer your greatest challenges, overcome daunting fears, or simply have enough energy to work a full-time job and still come home with a smile on your face and loving arms ready to hold your child and hear about her first day of kindergarten. And all the while, you'll be strutting your sexy stuff upon high, leg-flaunting heels. But only you can take yourself to the next level. You have to be accountable for your body.

*　*　*

Stop playing the victim! We don't play that game anymore. No matter which cards you have been dealt in life, you deserve happiness. You have the power to obtain that happiness if you take life by the horns and collect what is yours! Every second of each day is precious. Act like it. Take control and do something about your life and your body. It is no one else's responsibility but your own. Regardless of how imperfect or perfect you are, there is always room for improvement. Are you overweight, overstressed, overextended, and overtired? Believe it or not, exercise can help in every facet of your life. It will lift your mood, minimize your stress level, improve your sleep, cut your fat, increase your self-esteem, and tone your body and mind. Every single one of those changes will then radiate out and create more positive changes. When you are happy, those around you will be happier (have you ever heard the term "a smile is infectious?"). With less stress and better sleep, you will be able to think more clearly and make wise choices. Once your body slims, you will be able to fit in more flattering clothing, and your self-esteem will sky rocket, which can lead to any number of benefits—a raise, a new job, or a new partner.

How can you not put at least a little effort into attaining all of this greatness that lies latent within you? Get up and move your butt. Cut away some fat and make room for the new sexy and successful you!

> *It's not how many times you get knocked*
> *down, it is how many times you get back up.*
> —Vince Lombardi

You may be thinking, "Yeah, I already bought the books, went to the weekend fat-farm or confidence-building seminar; I followed the diets, lifted the weights, and punched the invisible bully, yet somehow I always failed." While there are a handful of really good trainers out there, the fact is that a lot of trainers and "exercise experts" got their personal training degrees at a weekend course— that's right, two days of training to be your personal trainer! Compare those two days to your lifetime of experience, during which you have spent endless hours testing out every fitness fad and diet phenomenon in hopes that one of them, any of them, would stick! Those other quick-fix gimmicks that you, and half the nation, got caught up with didn't help because A) they don't work or B) you didn't work (though it is probably a combination of the two). It is time to turn to a program that will work—and so will you.

> *Finish every day and be done with it. You have done what you could. Some blunders and absurdities no doubt have crept in; forget them as soon as you can. Tomorrow is a new day; begin it well and serenely and with too high a spirit to be cumbered with your old nonsense. This day is all that is good and fair. It is too dear, with its hopes and invitations, to waste a moment on yesterdays.*
>
> —Ralph Waldo Emerson

Now, don't get me wrong, many fitness plans do work—for a time. In fact, you may have had the opportunity to bask in the glow of weight-loss success for a short while. But as soon as you updated your wardrobe accordingly, inches inadvertently piled back on. And as the numbers on the scale began to climb, you were left feeling like a complete fitness failure. If your last fruitless slimming attempt included exercise, despite its shortcomings, I do applaud you for being on the right track. Regardless of which fitness routine rouses you, exercise is a good thing. But the problem often lies in the amount of time that you dedicate, each day, to that routine. Sure, you may lose weight doing 8 minutes here and 3 minutes there, but the reason that those programs often fail is because you don't feel good at the end of the routine. In fact, you may not feel anything at all, almost as if you never worked out in the first place. The sustained aerobic activity that you will experience with Cardio Barre will get your blood pumping, your heart racing, and your endorphins releasing. Endorphins, your body's nat-ural "feel good" chemicals, provide a natural, stress-relieving high immediately after your workout that continues throughout the day. And they are your key to long-term success.

Cardio Barre and this book are backed by decades of dance technique that have, until now, been coveted secrets of the industry. But, in order to achieve success, you have to embrace the lifestyle that comes with it. No, I am not talk-ing about endless auditions for Broadway shows. This is about tweaking your life in order to make room for the new you that you so badly want to reveal. Unless, of course, you enjoy throwing your time, money, and self-esteem into the bottomless pit of fruitless diets and workouts. I know, the process of change, the possibility of achieving the unknown, can be daunting, scary, frus-trating, and any other adjective that you want to throw into the pile. But that is because you are carrying around a lifetime supply of failure that has taught you to fear. Those other experts, diet books, exercise programs, and motivation tapes failed you in the past because you weren't taught how to *depend on your-self for your success.* You were led astray, by whatever trainer, nutritionist, or speaker whose spell you fell under. You looked to that person or that program for constant support and success instead of looking within yourself. After lean-ing on someone or something else for so long, you became dead weight, and you eventually fell. How many times have you fallen?

Well, now that you are entering my gym, leave your baggage and excuses outside and enter with the mind-set that you are ready for change. Once you re-alize that you hold the power, you will free yourself from your own restricting chains and release an unrelenting force from your depths. You will harness your newfound power and use your individual gifts to the best of your ability. You are ready to raise your bar.

It is time to stop compartmentalizing! Fitness should not be viewed as 45 min-utes of cardio followed by 20 minutes of strength training followed by 10 min-utes of stretching (if at all). Cardio Barre is the combination of cardio, strength training, and stretching in *one* no-impact, fast-paced, muscle trembling, fat-burning, body lengthening session. It is Pilates with a cardio burn, Tae Bo without the impact, ballet on hyperdrive with resistance. In short, Cardio Barre is a combination off all of the best elements of the most popular exercise programs, in one. The outcome? A long, lean, toned, strong, dancer-type body . . . the image of bodily perfection.

Celebrities are practically paid to be beautiful and trainers are often a daily occurrence, a way of life, a necessary component to their success. I know that your time is precious and hours dedicated to yourself are few and far between. Cardio Barre is designed to attain quick, yet long-term results for everyone. I have clients with such jam-packed schedules that they have less than 30 minutes a day to dedicate to themselves, let alone their workout. I have other clients who must train several hours a day in a short time span for demanding, time-crunched projects. Still other clients have endless leisure hours and exercise each day for the purpose of maintaining their already fit physiques. All I ask from you is that you make a commitment, not to me, but to yourself. Like I said before, I will provide the tools, but you have to put the tools to work.

Though some movements in Cardio Barre are minuscule, your muscles will be burning—Cardio Barre will bring awareness to *every* muscle in your body. You will walk around, going on with your day-to-day, *feeling* your body— sucking in your stomach, pulling your shoulders back, lifting your chest and your head. After a few sessions, you will notice your butt lifting and your waist tightening. You will feel excitement, wanting to begin your Cardio Barre program. After a few weeks you will see your muscles begin to pop, revealing definition and tone. You will notice your energy increasing, compliments and second glances boosting your self-esteem. You will exude self-confidence, radiance, composure, stamina, stability, grace, and you will finally feel comfortable in a bathing suit.

Despite all that I have said and all that you have read, I know the drill. . . . Some of you will actually read this book in its entirety, then put it down, sit on the couch with a bag of nachos, and continue living your sedentary life. I know your type. You are the same women or men who watch the Food Network for hours on end, then turn around and order takeout. For those of you who are even considering such insane inactivity, remember the age-old adage "move it or lose it." For some reason, many of you walk around with the misconception that you are immortal—until reality rears its dirty little head with the sudden death of a friend or family member, or when annually, as the new year passes, you realize you're another year older. Then you decide to "change your ways," frantically reorganizing your life as you take heed of your health and acknowledge the importance of your choices and their consequences. You find yourself sitting in the membership renewal office of your local gym and ordering workout videos like they're going out of style. The health food store becomes your new best friend, supplying you with whole grains, fruits, and vegetables to stock your refrigerator. You even up the ante by buying a brand-new exercise outfit to compliment your new attitude. But soon the severity of life fades and you accidentally fall back into your old routine. You feel too burdened to exercise and too exhausted to cook as you throw yourself on autopilot, awaiting the next jolting awakening, making you view life in a new light. Stop waiting for someone else's death to start your life! New Year's resolutions are not meant to be broken before you flip the calendar to February, folks! Get up and get going! Stop obsessing about your thighs and get on with your lives!

What is your happy weight? Approximately 75 percent of women admit that weight is always on their mind. Only about 15 percent of you consider your weight "just right." What is your internal monologue saying? No healthy change comes from self-loathing. Stop obsessing with the numbers on a scale. Why are you torturing yourself? If you are 35 and your goal weight is what it was when you were in high school, you are basically trying to hold a beach ball under water. Your happy weight should be what it is when you are in a happy state. That is what healthy is. Give yourself permission to be happy and healthy. It is time to move that gorgeous body of yours!

What I need you to do right now is ask yourself: What do you want? Who do you want to be? What does your mental picture of yourself look like right now? What do you want it to look like? If you want it bad enough, you have got to raise the barre. You have to own up to who you are and how you feel right now: fat, uninspired, insecure, clumsy, whatever you may be, and be prepared to change that about yourself. You have got to want it so badly that you can taste it, that you can visualize yourself in that body, that mind-set, that new you. You have to free yourself from unhealthy emotional attachments and self-sabotaging habits. You have to reach so deep within yourself that it will hurt. You may have to break yourself down in order to put yourself back together the way you want to be seen, the way you want to feel. This will be harder than a kickboxing class, more intense than a ten-mile run. Sometimes the toughest thing to do is look yourself in the face and own the image that you have created. Regular exercise classes will open your body, and maybe even your mind, but it is opening your heart that can be the most torturous.

He who would leap far must first take a long run.
—DANISH PROVERB

If you are ready, let's do this. I will be here, as your personal trainer, every day. I will drag you out of bed if I have to, stick with you through pain, encourage you through weakness, and be the first to congratulate you during each achievement, every step of the way. The fact is, you can't afford not to do this workout—for the sake of your health. I will guide you through the 8 weeks to your perfect body. I will help you to rouse motivation that will start you on this new path toward perfection. So grab the barre and hold on for dear life.

1

3 Key Elements of Fitness

Fitness is not just about running (cardio), lifting weights (strength training), or yoga (flexibility). According to the American Council on Exercise (ACE), in order to have a complete workout, it is essential to incorporate all three elements. Lucky for you, the three key elements to any fitness program—cardio, resistance, and flexibility—are each woven throughout every Cardio Barre workout.

Cardio

If you want to burn fat and slim down, you have to do cardio. No, I am not telling you to run a 5k in order to get your heart rate up. We have no use for shin splints or blisters. Running often leads exercisers to get off on the wrong foot. Do you know how many women tell me they don't do cardio because they don't like running? There are other ways to get your heart pumping; Cardio Barre is one of them.

While walking is a cardio activity, this low-intensity workout effectively, but slowly, burns body fat. What does that mean? The intensity is the level at which your heart and breathing rate are elevated for a sustained period of time. Cardio Barre, on the other hand, is a high-intensity exercise, which has been said to burn body fat 9 times faster than low intensity exercises. After a high-intensity workout, once the music stops and cool down begins, hormones that were released during your workout take over and continue to burn fat and calories for several hours! What could be better than not working out and still burning calories?

More than burning fat, studies show that a high-intensity cardio session has several health benefits including:

- Dramatically boosts the metabolism both during and after the workout
- Body fat is more readily transformed into energy, which is exerted during a workout
- Considerable increase in aerobic capacity, stamina, and strength
- Mental and physical stress and tension reduction
- Increased and sustained energy
- Improved sleep
- Strengthened heart and lungs
- More efficient use of oxygen
- Increased circulation
- Reduced risk of some cancers
- Reduced risk of heart disease
- Lower blood pressure
- Longer life

Strength Training

No, lifting a few light weights, and even a heavy one here and there (like your own body weight during push-ups), will not turn you into a muscle-bound meathead. When strength training, men develop muscles differently than women. Men will usually get bigger by increasing muscle fiber size, while women get stronger by using a higher percentage of muscle fibers. I know, many of you may still have a stigma against lifting weights, in fear that it will de-feminize you. But, believe me, it will only make you sexier. The unfortunate myth originated centuries ago when sports (particularly strength-driven) were designated as male-only activities. Finally, in the 1950s, women began to in-corporate strength training into their workout routines to help improve their performance and athleticism in track and field. Though times have changed, the strength-training stigma sometimes persists. With few, if any, exceptions, female athletes today depend on strength training to be on top of their game. And, according to studies, 94 percent of athletes do not feel as though their strong musculature and athletic lifestyles makes them feel less feminine. They beautifully balance strength and femininity.

Women who strength train feel empowered. The ability to attempt and overcome daunting physical challenges, as well as to increase strength and mus-cle definition, make women feel as though they are the master of their domain, and that they can protect their own temple, without the help of a man, thank you very much! So why are women feeling so strong and in control? Because they are. Strength training helps trim fat and increase lean muscle. This re-composition may result in a slight gain of scale weight, but that is only because muscle weighs more than fat. Regardless of weight in pounds, inches are what matter. When you lose fat and gain muscle, you lose inches, especially in the lower body. You may notice a slight increase in girth in your upper body as your twiggy arms gain a little muscular definition. But, in general, unless you have a genetic predisposition to gain a lot of muscle mass, or you are doing high-weight, high-intensity weight lifting (which you won't be doing in Cardio Barre), you will decrease in size.

The fact is that having a little muscle will actually help you burn more fat and create that lean, svelte feminine physique that you want. Strength training is what actually reshapes your body—creating tone and sculpting you sexy! The more muscle you have (again, I am not talking about bulky muscles), the faster your metabolism will be, the more calories and fat you will naturally burn . . . even while you sleep. Why? Well, muscle tissue is very active in nature. In order to maintain itself, one pound of muscle burns about 35 calories a day! Without you having to lift a weight. This is why having muscle will help you stay slim. As

Fit Tip

Flabby muscles: The real cause of flabby muscles is lack of exercise, not aging. Muscle mass does decline between the ages of 30 and 70. But isotonic-strength-building exercises can reverse the decline. Isotonic exercise, which includes calisthenics and weight lifting, is the contraction and relaxation of muscles, causing the muscle to shorten and lengthen. Half an hour of isotonics 2 or 3 times a week can increase strength within 2 weeks and double it in 12 weeks—by changing the ratio of muscle to fat. Bonus: isotonics increases bone density, helping prevent bone fractures caused by osteoporosis.

you lose muscle, your metabolism loses steam, making it harder to lose and keep weight off.

Studies have shown that one of the main reasons why yo-yo dieters are, well, yo-yo dieters is because of muscle loss. When calories are drastically cut, weight quickly falls off. But up to 25 percent of that weight is actually muscle tissue, which, as we just discussed, helps the body naturally burn fat. So, in the end, you are actually doing your diet a disservice when you lose muscle.

Incorporating strength training into your workout can benefit your body because it:

- Fortifies more than just your muscles, as your bones and connective tissue are strengthened as well. Osteoporosis is a major concern for women these days. Increasing bone density through strength training can minimize your risk of osteoporosis.
- After age 20, the average adult loses a half pound of muscle tissue each year. Remember, less muscle tissue means fewer calories burned.
- Life seems less strenuous when you are strong. Daily routines and tasks like carrying groceries and pushing a baby carriage are easier to do when you have strength of your side.

Ninety million Americans have fallen into the anti-aging web of products and procedures. Yes, burning fat and increasing strength are certainly reasons to lift weights, but more than for the aesthetic value, strength training has been proven to assist in slowing the physiological clock—yes, lifting weights can help with anti-aging! It is all part of the exercise equation: cardio exercise maintains the heart and lungs, while strength training maintains the muscles and bones. Don't leave it out.

Flexibility

Ever hear of Flex Appeal? I'm not asking you to go Gumby. You don't have to be a gymnast to be sufficiently flexible. But can you bend over and touch your toes? You may have been able to touch your toes and then some when you were younger, but it is just as important, or more, to be flexible when you begin to add a few years to your life. Yes, that is the kind and gentle way of saying, as you age. Each passing year, your muscles and joints lose a little bit of their range of motion. Your tendons begin to shorten and tighten. To compensate, posture loses its straight stance. After a few years, each little bit adds up to a lot, hindering your active lifestyle and day-to-day activities. Being limber allows you to utilize your body to its fullest, even as gray hairs begin to grow on your head.

No, stretching doesn't aid in weight loss, and I realize that to some, it can be a boring, tedious, slow-moving task. But stretching and increasing flexibility has rewards that far outweigh the frustration and boredom of the activity itself. Do you want long and lean or short and bulky muscles? Stretching literally stretches the muscles, lengthening them (again, think of a dancer's legs) until they are long and lean and sexy! While lengthening your muscles, you are also shortening your recovery time, minimizing painful tightening and gripping of the muscles after an intense workout. In order to avoid the time-consuming post-workout pause of stretching, in Cardio Barre, I created a workout that includes stretching throughout the workout itself.

More than allowing you to be able to do the splits, flexibility lends itself to a long list of benefits, including:

- Maintains your body's range of motion
- Helps prevent injury during exercise and daily activity

- Allows for a moment to relax both the body and mind
- Encourages the development of body awareness
- Promotes circulation
- Improves posture

The 8 Core Elements of Cardio Barre

Posture and Body Awareness

A characteristic way of bearing one's body; carriage. A frame of mind affecting one's thoughts or behavior; an overall attitude.

Your posture is the physical manifestation of your inner state. Once established as a pattern, neuromuscular tension reinforces your awkward stance and, in an attempt to correct the imbalance, bones develop to fortify the curvature. Soon, like the chicken and the egg, you may forget which came first—insecurity due to a hunched back, or a hunched back due to insecurity. Thankfully, you can increase confidence and straighten your stance through exercise. I will teach you how to hold your shoulders back, lift your chest, and develop a physique that exudes self-esteem. Supportive muscles will soon develop around your neck, chest, shoulders, and back, to hold the newly constructed confident you in place! Because posture is the core of self-esteem, it is a core of Cardio Barre. After a few sessions with me, your butt will lift, your chest will lift, and your mood will lift.

Core

The basic or most important part; the essence. The center or innermost part.

Experts are finally beginning to understand the importance of core strength—something dancers have known for hundreds of years. Your core is your "center," and everything radiates from the center . . . so when your center is strengthened, everything else will follow. Core strength will improve posture and back problems, which are very common and usually attributed to a weak abdomen. When engaged, your core can assist in almost every movement, minimizing unnecessary strain. Why tense your neck within an exercise when you can tense your belly instead, therefore adding another muscle to your workout? I base every exercise on core strength, so you are always working your abs—not just during crunches. You may be focused on your arms, but your core will also be activated. When you lift your leg, you better believe that your tummy will be tight. This leads, again, to more control and heightened overall awareness. When you get in touch with stimulating your core, you will start to feel it engage before anything else. You will find that you are strengthening and lengthening your center at the same time, a principle often used in Pilates. You can test this by doing a simple push-up, or even just by pushing against a wall gently. You will notice that the abdomen will engage before your upper-body primary muscles. You have reached your core!

Balance

The ability to keep one's body steady without falling.

Balance is the key to a happy life. Whether we are talking about food, fitness, work, or relationships, the recurrent theme that seems to surface time and time again is balance. When it comes to your body, balance is also essential in your day-to-day activities. It is something we strive for from the moment we, as babies, flip from our back to our bellies and learn to crawl. Soon we muster enough confidence to attempt to stand, then walk. Now that you have mastered that art, balance is less about falling and more about staying properly aligned. When you experience pain or weakness in your body, you are out of balance. To accommodate tension in your shoulders, you may be placing unnecessary strain on your neck. If your right ankle is broken, your left knee may take the brunt of your energy, causing it to be next in line to give way. Striving constantly to be in balance, the body naturally compensates for weakness. This can actually be used toward your advantage. If you live with discomfort or pain, you can reduce or eliminate it by learning how to strengthen smaller supportive muscles, allowing the weakness to heal. Maintaining proper alignment and bodily balance will help you maintain a healthier body longer.

Opposition

Exactly in reverse or in contrast.

Cardio Barre constantly focuses on working the body in opposite directions at the same time to lengthen, elongate, and lift. It is the secret to a ballerina's strong stance and a tree's dominating presence—imagine your roots growing down as yours branches soar upward. Too whimsical for you? Picture an invisible string that is attached to the very top of your head, and imagine someone pulling that string tight, elongating your neck, creating space between your ears and your shoulders and lengthening your spine. When you "Plie," a move that you will soon be quite familiar with, you may be squatting down, but you must think of lifting your torso and head up. This is the secret to lengthening and elongating at the same time, giving you a longer leaner appearance and better posture.

Press/Push/Pull

To reshape or make compact by applying steady force; compress. A vigorous or insistent effort toward an end. To stretch (taffy, for example) repeatedly, to apply force to so as to cause or tend to cause motion toward the source of the force.

By eliminating "punch" and "kick," and replacing them with "press," "push," and "pull," I have created a no-impact workout that applies little stress to joints while strengthening the supportive muscles surrounding them. When you press, push, or pull, you are working with resistance without submitting your muscles and joints to unnecessary damage. This affords the muscles the ability to work safely yet effectively. Steady, nonexplosive movements are particularly ideal for people with back, knee, hip, and joint problems, as well as for pregnant women. And if you are lucky enough not to experience any such pain, no-impact exercise will help you avoid it in the future.

Stretch

To draw out to full length, to a greater size or distance.

Don't just stretch at the end of a workout. To ensure a safe workout and help avoid injury, stretch after your warm-up, but before your workout, when your muscles are warm and pliable. Stretching before a warm-up, when muscles are still cold, is not safe. Like a frozen rubber band, they can snap. Yes, you heard me right, DO NOT stretch until you are sufficiently warmed up. Bending a cold body over to touch your toes in an attempt of "warming" up your muscles is doing little more than testing your tendon's ability to stay intact. A warm rubber band, on the other hand, can easily elongate when gently stretched. Stretching at the end of a workout keeps the muscles elongated and helps to prevent from bulking up. It also aids in recovery time and helps avoid soreness. Also, as you get older, your muscles get shorter, making daily chores more difficult. Stretching will improve your way of life and make getting around and doing daily activities easier. More than before and after, Cardio Barre incorporates stretching throughout the entire exercise routine so that you are constantly strengthening and stretching. Stretching also helps with blood circulation, aiding in the reduced appearance of cellulite and varicose veins. Psychologically, stretching allows you to slow down, take some quiet time, and de-stress. It will relax those muscle and mental tensions and help you to calm yourself, both physically and emotionally. Remember, we are striving for the long lean look of a dancer. Stretching helps muscles get longer and appear leaner.

Squeeze

Contracting by applying force.

The difference between "activity" and "productivity" is that in an activity you go through the motion aimlessly, but with productivity, you make the effort count. Make your movement productive and you will get results. By squeezing a muscle while you work, and not just placing it into the next position, you will maximize the stress on the muscle, therefore creating a constantly productive movement. Time and energy are tight and in demand, so don't waste any. Concentrating on the squeeze, during both the contraction and release, creates an efficient, natural resistance without the use of weights. In order to create that weighty contraction, imagine what it would feel like to be holding a 5-, 10-, even 50-pound free weight in your hand. Believe it or not, the mind is a very powerful tool, with the ability to create resistance when no physical resistance is actually present. With this constant working movement, you will burn more calories and fat, while gaining more strength more quickly.

Isolate

To set apart from the others.

A typical aerobics class will work the major muscle groups. Cardio Barre isolates the smaller muscle groups that most other fitness routines miss, while simultaneously working the major muscle groups. This isolation allows you to maintain constant control of your body's movements, avoiding the injury-inducing flailing of limbs. For injured and pregnant exercisers, isolation can allow you to keep up your fitness program by avoiding certain untouchable areas. Overall, isolation enables you to shape, sculpt, define, and reduce certain spots on your body like never before.

2

3 Keys to Maintaining Optimum Health

Obesity is currently the second most preventable cause of death in the United States (smoking still ranks as number one). This growing problem has generated so much attention lately that the topic has even secured frequent front-page headlines and feature stories on traditionally politically driven magazines, newspapers, and national television news shows. On the cover of a recent issue of *The Economist,* the evolution of man was portrayed in an illustration depicting the progression from an ape to a fat man sipping a supersize soda, and the magazine's headline read, "The Shape of Things to Come." In this diet-obsessed nation, why are we so fat? To slim our sprawling waistlines there are three key ingredients: exercise, diet, and rest.

Exercise

According to the Center for Disease Control (CDC), healthy adults should do at least 30 minutes of moderate to vigorous exercise 5 or more days per week for optimum health. In order to attain maximum health benefits from your workouts, it is important to include the 3 key elements of fitness: cardio, strength training, and flexibility.

The 1996 Surgeon General's report *Physical Activity and Health* recognized that moderate physical activity has the ability to significantly decrease the risk of developing or dying from heart disease, diabetes, colon cancer, and high blood pressure. In general, physically active people live longer lives of higher quality than inactive people.

This quality of life is abundantly clear when you look at the statistics, the scientific proof, and doctors' opinions suggesting that physical activity helps prevent the leading cause of death in America—coronary heart disease. Some studies say that physically inactive people have double the risk of developing heart disease compared to active people. In addition to heart disease, inactive people increase their chances of developing high blood pressure, high cholesterol, obesity, and even picking up a smoking habit! Do you know how many drugs are developed to combat these often self-inflicted ailments? Just turn on the TV and you will be bombarded with ads from drug companies who promise to reduce these effects of inactivity, when all you have to do is exercise and avoid them in the first place! Avoiding life-threatening disease can be so simple.

Exercise is especially important for people who suffer from joint or bone pain. Twenty percent of adults have arthritis—yet on average, regardless of exercise's promise to better your body and ease ailments, they remain less active than people without arthritis. Flexibility, strength training, and cardiovascular activity have been shown to help arthritis sufferers preserve normal joint mobility, improve muscle flexibility and strength, and, in turn, support weak joints while protecting them from further damage. Exercise helps arthritis patients maintain or reduce weight, therefore alleviating pressure placed on joints; it maintains the strength and health of bone and cartilage tissue and increases endurance and cardiovascular fitness in order to oxygenate the blood and strengthen the heart and lungs. More than 25 million people suffer from the chronic condition of osteoporosis, an often unnecessary and possibly reversible condition if only sufferers would partake in regular physical activity, including strength training, to increase bone density. Stop the excuses of "oh my back hurts" or "but my joints are stiff today," and move your body. The fact of the matter is that your joints are likely stiff because you are not putting them to use. Your connective tissues and muscles are becoming atrophied and deteriorating as you become more and more sedentary. Exercising will improve your physical state. It will strengthen your muscles, make your connective tissues more malleable, and minimize pains and strains. Unless your doctor recommends otherwise, there is a good chance that exercise will decrease pain, lessen stiffness, and increase mobility.

If you have never exercised a day in your life, and the prospect of starting something new seems too daunting, but you want to be healthier, you are beginning from a great place, because the only place you can go is up! Isn't that a great feeling? As long as you do *something* to move your body, you have already succeeded! You don't have to jump into an intense daily workout routine immediately. Ease into it. I bet that after a few sessions you will find that you feel so good that you can hardly imagine giving up now! But give yourself more than just the first day; promise me that. Mounting studies suggest that even moderate physical activity can make major changes to your quality of life. Starting a new program, which requires time, also requires a little reorganizing of your regular routine in order to fit this addition in. Once you figure out how to incorporate exercise into your life, making it another one of your routines—like walking your dog or making pancakes on Sundays—it will be easy to keep up.

Benefits of Exercise
> Reduces or maintains body weight and fat percentage
> Builds and maintains muscles, bones, and joints
> Reduces depression and anxiety
> Improves psychological well-being
> Increases self-esteem and confidence
> Enhances work, recreation, and sport performance
> Reduces the risk of premature death
> Reduces the risk of heart disease
> Reduces high blood pressure
> Reduces high cholesterol

Reduces the risk of colon and breast cancer

Reduces the risk of developing diabetes

While the benefits of physical activity are proven to improve and lengthen life, according to the CDC, more than 50 percent of American adults neglect to get enough exercise to reap its rewards. In fact, of those 50 percent, half are completely inactive during their leisure time. Unfortunately, Americans are not hearing, or not listening, to the constant onslaught of information on exercise's benefits, considering that only about 23 percent of adults in the United States engage in intense physical activity at least three times per week for the minimum suggested 20 minutes per session. Only 15 percent of adults living in the United States follow the suggested workout recommendation of 5 days a week or more for 30 minutes or longer per session. If that fact isn't depressing enough, of that huge percentage of inactive Americans, the majority of them are women. Ladies, it is time to move your butts. You may want to get your kids moving right along with you, considering that more than a third of children in 9th through 12th grade do not exercise vigorously, and that their activity levels are dropping every year.

In an attempt to increase the amount of exercisers, a group of scientists, both inside and outside of the government, got together and determined the health priorities and feasible objectives that this country could tackle in the near future. In January 2000 they published a set of healthy goals called Healthy People 2010. Two overarching, ultimate objectives were determined: (1) Increase life expectancy and quality of life. (2) Eliminate health disparities. Twenty-eight areas of focus were established. And of the 29 health issues that Healthy People 2010 believes are important to this country, physical activity is listed as number one. Breaking those twenty-eight areas of focus down into individual goals, in order to better our lives, 467 initiatives were created in total. Among other things, Healthy People hopes that by 2010 the proportion of adults who engage in regular, if not daily, physical activity in general increases. In addition, Healthy People aims to see an increase in individual strength, endurance, and flexibility activities. We are almost at the 2010 deadline. How close are you to achieving your fitness goals? It is time to raise your bar!

Statistics and facts are all pretty serious. So, to lighten up the mood, let's talk about sex. More than a means of achieving a shapely physique, several studies point to the possibility that exercise can reignite a dull sex life. According to a study reported in the *Journal of the American Medical Association* (*JAMA*), sexual dysfunction is more common in people with poor physical health than those who exercise regularly. Other studies have found that those who exercise regularly have intercourse more frequently and enjoy more orgasms. Why? Well, doctors suspect that one reason for the increase in sexual pleasure is that exercise promotes good circulation, which promotes sexual function. Exercise triggers the release of endorphins, the same chemicals that are released from "aphrodisiac" foods such as chocolate, stimulating a euphoric state. If for nothing else, for the sake of your sex life, exercise!

Diet

Eating a healthy diet is essential to maintaining a healthy body. What determines a healthy diet is rooted in food choice and portion size. The idea is not quantity over quality; it is quality over quantity. Again, health is about balance. Unfortunately, diet is where many weight-loss programs falter. Counting calories, measuring portions, avoiding this, restricting that, it can all get very confusing. Confusion results in frustration, which, in turn, results in giving up, throwing in the towel, forgetting about your newfound healthy lifestyle and going back to your old, easier ways of mindless eating. Try to eat healthier, higher quality foods. Instead of mindlessly scarfing down spoonfuls of food, hardly tasting the flavors before they are at the back of your throat and swallowed, savor each bite as you chew. If you want to splurge *once* in a while, you can. But have three bites of a super rich fudge brownie instead of an entire pan of low-fat chocolate cake. The tasteless calories you consume when you eat a low-fat cake do not even come close to measuring up to the fewer calories you ingest with a few flavor-filled bites!

To help you make healthier choices, take a look at the food pyramid. Yes, it is that triangle that appears on the side of cereal boxes and the wrapping of packaged bread. It is time to finally pay it a little attention. The food pyramid lays out nutrition facts in a very easy-to-understand, visual way. It is a guide, and it should be yours.

In late 2004 the pyramid went under scrutiny by the U.S. Department of Agriculture (USDA). In an attempt to battle the bulge that much of America has succumbed to, plans for a new pyramid addressed individual lifestyles in addition to the suggested servings of fruits, vegetables, grains, and meats. Because the exact size of a serving seemed somewhat nebulous to the average consumer, there were thoughts of translating servings into actual hard amounts, suggesting cups and ounces instead of "servings."

Finally, in April 2005, in hopes of making consumers take more notice of the nutritional icon, the USDA launched a new pyramid dubbed the MyPyramid food guidance system. This is the first time, since 1992, that the pyramid has been tinkered with, creating a more updated, user friendly version that turned the triangle on its side. Instead of the old pyramid with divided horizontal boxes suggesting serving sizes, the new MyPyramid features colorful vertical stripes in varying thickness, each representing a specific food group. In addition to the six bands of colors corresponding to food groups, along the pyramid's side is a staircase and a runner treading up the hill, illuminating the importance of exercise to achieve optimum health. In the same breath, use the pyramid only as a guide, not as a strict set of rules that should be followed to the letter. Of the six dietary guidelines, three of them are really key: (1) Balance and variety is essential. (2) Eat plenty of fruits, vegetables, and grains. (3) Keep fat and sugar to a minimum.

Healthier choices to consider:

Fiber and Carbohydrates

Carbohydrates should not be considered the "c" word, shunned from your pantry and crossing the threshold of your mouth only on very special occasions. Contrary to popular food fads out there, the best diets focus on healthy carbohydrates and fiber. Stop the ban on whole grains, breads, rice, cereals, and pasta. Starch is not fattening. Calories and fat add fat. Of course, if consuming a heaping plate full of pasta that is bigger than the size of your head is a daily practice—yes, you will gain weight. But that's because you are eating enough for five people. Do you know how many calories are in that oversized serving? Add cream sauce and you've just eaten the equivalent of a birthday cake. Come on now, diet is about balance—no cutting entire food groups out and gorging yourself on others.

There is a difference between simple carbohydrates and fiber-filled carbohydrates. You want the second one; in fact, you want a lot of it. Throw away the white bread and fill your fridge with multigrain bread. I realize that there is currently a no-carbohydrate frenzy, causing hoards of people to ditch healthy carbohydrates, filled with nutrient-rich, appetite-curbing fiber. The diet dilemma can be confusing, I know. But this food group fight is doing nothing but making us neglect essential dietary elements. We have just emerged from an era that demonized fat. In an attempt to extricate any sign of the enemy, fat was eliminated from numerous common foods, including cakes and cookies! The end result was a nation of carbohydrate-loaded dieters who supplemented steak for pasta and one regular cookie for ten of the fat-free version. In hopes of reversing what was quickly rounding out to be an epidemic of overweight people, other extreme diets were created that cut out various elemental necessities from our daily food regimens. This latest craze of cutting carbohydrates, like fat-free diets, too shall pass. There is no one category of foods that is good or bad. The challenge is trying to figure out which are better and which are worse. Fiber-filled complex carbohydrates is the better carb.

Did your mom ever tell you it was important to eat your "roughage?" Why? Because roughage keeps you regular. What garnered lettuce, cruciferous vegetables like broccoli, and fruit the name "roughage?" Fiber. Along with grains, vegetables are naturally filled with fiber. Foods that are rich in fiber help clean out the digestive track, keeping everything running smoothly—through you and out of you. In fact, the main ingredient in many natural laxatives is psyllium husk, one of the best sources of fiber. Because of its laxative effect, fiber helps with weight management.

High-fiber foods are bulky, yet they contain few calories since they are made up of indigestible plant products. If your body can't break it down and digest it, your body also can't consume its calories. Fiber quickly fills you up, curbing your appetite. It is slow to digest, preventing spikes in blood sugar levels. Because it is such a slow-moving, bulky mass as it travels through your digestive tract, it helps to flush out residual waste and toxins from fatty, stickier foods that previously made their way through your system and stuck to the walls of your intestines on their way out. More than its laxative effects, fiber has been known to help reduce the risk of obesity, type II diabetes, cardiovascular disease, high cholesterol, and certain types of cancer. So why aren't you eating your fair share of this health-promoting food? According to statistics, most Americans get only about 10 to 12 grams of fiber per day, but the recommended daily dose is between 30 and 35 grams per day. In order to reap fiber's benefits, you have got to at least double your intake. Be aware that, since fiber is so filling, it has been known to bloat and cause gastrointestinal distress when consumed in high quantities. Balance, remember that.

Bottom line: You are likely eating much less fiber than you should. So up your amount!

Protein

According to the MyPyramid food guide suggestion for protein intake, you are likely eating way too much of it! The pyramid recommends that you bake, broil, or grill low-fat or lean meats, or poultry (this means chicken, turkey, and other birds), plus fish, beans, eggs, tofu, tempeh, or nuts for variation *each day*. Notice that the protein portion of the guide is much less than the grains portion, therefore, you should be eating less protein and more grains each day.

Protein does not necessarily mean bacon and fried chicken. Lean protein can help you shed those unwanted pounds and keep your belly full. Protein can be very good for you, but it is important to choose lean meats and lower fat dairy products to minimize unnecessary fat intake. Think of it as one of your body's main fuel sources. Unlike sugar's energetic instant gratification effect (which quickly burns away, leaving you with less energy than you started with), protein provides long-lasting energy that, along with complex carbohydrates, helps make you feel full while steadying blood sugar levels and staving off hunger until your next snack or meal. Take notice of my mention of carbohydrates, along with protein. Despite what many protein-heavy diets may promote, you should not attempt to sustain yourself on protein alone. Balance is key to any long-term health and weight-loss success.

In addition to energy, protein is a rich source of iron in your diet. There are times in your life, for example during your menstrual cycle, when it would be a good idea to up your protein intake in order to increase the amount of iron in your body. Especially for women of childbearing age, your period results in a large amount of blood loss, which can lead to iron deficiency. Pregnancy is another period in your life when an increase in iron is recommended.

If you are a vegetarian, you need to pay extra attention to getting enough protein in your diet. When it comes to iron, you primarily will need to focus on spinach, chard, beans, lentils, and peas, which are all naturally high in iron. For those of you with an aversion to spinach and chard, thankfully, most processed grains—including cereals, pasta, and bread—are fortified with iron.

Even if you are getting a sufficient amount of iron in your diet, it isn't all necessarily being absorbed; this is a prime example of why we need to eat well-balanced meals. Vitamin C assists the body in the absorption of iron. I know, you may be thinking that this whole iron conversation is not that important in the grand scheme of your diet, but women who are iron deficient can become anemics, which can result in fatigue, dizziness, irritability, and headaches. If you feel like fainting, there is a good chance you won't be exercising.

Bottom line: eat a balanced amount of lean protein.

Fruits and Vegetables

Fruits and vegetables should be more than garnish or dashes of color on your plate. A healthy plate should be doused in color—reds, greens, *and* oranges! Eat 5 servings of fruits and vegetables daily to minimize the risk of cardiovascular disease and cancer. Dark-colored fruits and vegetables generally contain more vitamins and nutrients than light-colored options. To get all the goodness out of your veggies, choose fresh or frozen over canned.

Aside from the grains section of the food guide system, the fruit and vegetable sections are two of the more ignored groups. Some of you may make excuses as to why you aren't eating enough fruits and veggies, attempting to convince yourself that they are inconvenient. Yet I don't remember the last time

I saw someone pull a chicken breast out of their coat pocket and start snacking. Fruits and vegetables are probably the most convenient of all of your food choices. Yeah, broccoli may taste a little better (to some) when cooked, but cooking is not essential in order to eat it. Fruits and vegetables are truly the original fast food. Come on now, if you are looking for convenience, grab a banana, or throw an apple or tangerine into your purse. Too messy? How about some carrot sticks or dried cranberries. Enough excuses! Eat your fruits and veggies!

According to the MyPyramid food guide, you are not eating enough servings of vegetables or fruit! Are you? It is suggested that you eat more dark green vegetables, more orange vegetables, more dried peas and beans, and a variety of fruits—that includes fresh, frozen, canned, and dry fruit. Notice a trend? MORE! Eat *more* fruits and veggies.

The food guide is not just there to be a thorn in your behind. There are reasons why it is recommended to eat certain amounts of certain foods. The reason is your health. In fact, the U.S. Department of Health and Human Services, the U.S. Department of Agriculture, and the National Academy of Sciences have all conducted studies to determine the impact of fruits and vegetables on our bodies. What they discovered is that eating a diet filled with fruits and vegetables, in addition to low-fat, low-cholesterol, whole-grain foods, may have the potential to decrease your risk of developing heart disease and cancer.

Fruit and vegetables, as a whole, are food groups brimming with healing properties. But other studies have been done to figure out the benefits of individual fruits and veggies. It has been discovered that the antioxidant properties of grapes may help reduce levels of blood fat such as cholesterol. Grape skins themselves are filled with pterostilbene and resveratrol (the chemical cousins of antioxidants), which have been shown to have cancer-fighting and anti-inflammatory effects. To help hinder the spread of breast cancer, chew a few heads of broccoli. Even eye-watering onions have proved themselves worthy of healing praise! They contain certain compounds that can slow the spread of cancer. Onion's equally pungent friend garlic has been linked to a decreased risk of breast cancer. The fuzzy kiwi fruit is filled with the antioxidant vitamin C and can help with anti-aging by minimizing macular degeneration and decreasing your risk of eye diseases such as cataracts. Another hearty antioxidant that fills several of our favorite fruits is lycopene. National news shows have reported stories that lycopene may help protect men from prostate cancer by slowing tumor growth in the prostate. Women benefit from it too. Lycopene is a red-tinted compound found in tomatoes (the highly publicized healthy fruit), red watermelon, and guava. So what is so great about lycopene? Studies suggest that it may be able to boost heart health and prevent heart disease.

The nutritional goodness of fruits and vegetables is undeniable. Unless stir-fried with loads of oil, dipped in butter, or baked in a pie, they are naturally low in calories and fat. Of course, there are a few exceptions, including avocados, coconuts, and olives, but those fats are naturally "good fats." Fruits and vegetables are loaded with vitamins A and C, filled with fiber, and often folate and vitamin B (especially peas and dried beans) and some are sweet as candy. A handful of fresh or frozen strawberries and blueberries, and you have got yourself a delicious and healthy dessert!

Fat

More so than carbohydrates, fat has historically, or at least in recent history, been slapped with "F-word" status. Yes, we are in the midst of emerging from an era that demonized fat. In an attempt to extricate any sign of the enemy, fat was eliminated from numerous common foods, including cakes and cookies! The end result was a nation of dieters who ate so many carbs that they raised their blood sugar and got fat. In fact, Americans have become so afraid of getting fat that we have leached any sign of that nasty "F" word from our lives (except when we sneak a cookie when no one is looking, but that doesn't count, right?). In hopes of reversing what was quickly rounding out to be an epidemic of overweight people, other extreme diets were created that cut out various elemental necessities from our daily food regimens. Some of those diets promoted mass consumption of the thing we fear most—*fat*! It is time to even out in order to drop weight.

Clearly there is a lot of confusion around what to eat and what not to eat because, somehow, our waistlines continue to expand. Considering the enormous attention we place on health, dieting, and exercise, it is truly shocking how big we have become. Sadly, America is more obese than it has ever been. In 2004,

Health and Human Services secretary Tommy Thompson acknowledged obesity as a huge problem that has become even more than a personal concern—it is a public health concern. He unveiled a national education campaign encouraging Americans to begin to take small steps to fight obesity. More than encouragement, he released a new obesity research strategy at the National Institutes of Health. Obese Americans are suffering too much and dying too young. In January 2004 the journal *Obesity Research* reported that obesity-related health costs now account for a large portion of total health care spending. In 2003, Americans foot the bill for approximately $75 billion on obesity-related health care, from heart disease and cancer to diabetes. If we continue growing at the rate we have been, that figure is expected to almost double by 2015! Why are we having so much trouble controlling our ever-expanding bodies? One reason is that we have been jumping around from one fad diet to the next, constantly shocking our metabolisms. Another reason is that we are simply eating too much fat. Why? Unfortunately, fat tastes good. From cookies and cakes to chicken wings and cheese, we seem to constantly be stuffing our faces with fat. Stop! Life is more important than those five minutes of taste-bud fulfillment.

Thankfully, all fat is not bad for you. There are even fats that are called "good fats," and they are absolutely essential elements to your diet. Put away the potato chips and start eating some healthy fat. Seriously.

Good fats are naturally occurring dietary polyunsaturated fats that we find in fruits such as avocados, coconuts, and olives (olive oil). Good fats are also in grains, seeds, nuts, and beans like flaxseed, almonds, and soybeans. Yes, nuts are good! In recent years, people have been going nuts about nuts. Sorry, I had to say it. They may be high in fat, but the benefits outweigh the negatives. You want proof? Scientists at Harvard School of Public Health found that women who consumed a serving of nuts or a half serving of peanut butter 5 times per week had a 30 percent lower chance of acquiring "adult onset" or type II diabetes. Other studies have revealed that almonds, walnuts, and pecans can increase heart health and lower LDL cholesterol (bad cholesterol). Eating as few as 8 to 10 walnuts per day has been shown to help prevent the hardening of arteries. Preliminary tests with brazil nuts have suggested that they can lower breast-cancer risk. Recent research has revealed that the omega-3 fatty acids in walnuts can help minimize the build up of plaque in the arteries. Eating a handful of vitamin E–rich almonds has been linked to the reduction of the risk of bladder cancer.

But it's not just nuts that you need to add more of to your diet. Fish has been shown to be very healthy too. Fish, especially cold-water fish like salmon, trout, striped bass, mackerel, herring, and sardines, are filled with omega-3 fatty acids, a type of good fat. What makes omega-3 so great? Scientists have shown that people who eat a diet high in omega-3 fatty acids reduce their risk of heart disease, cancer, obesity, and diabetes, while minimizing the pain of arthritis and improving their moods. These benefits have been seen in people who eat cold-water fish twice weekly.

According to our trusty food guide pyramid, you should eat fats and sweets sparingly. But don't forget that fat naturally occurs in meat, poultry, fish, some fruits, vegetables, and grains. In general, fat should make up about 20 percent of your total daily caloric intake. Fat has a high concentration of calories, but don't completely leave it out of your diet. It is a major source of fuel for your body. Look at it as energy stored beneath your skin. Without at least some fat, your body does not function properly. It insulates you, keeping you protected from the cold. Fat also cushions your organs, provides energy, helps make up certain hormones, keeps your skin and hair healthy, and maintains and transports fat-soluble vitamins A, D, E, and K throughout your body. In fact, fat is present in every living cell of your body.

Now that I have gone on and on about the importance of fat, it is even more important that you know the differences between different types of fat. Like carbohydrates (white bread versus whole wheat), there are good fats and not so good fats. While it is important to eat the good fats, it is also important not to eat the bad fats, or else you will get fat.

There are three main types of dietary fat: polyunsaturated, monounsaturated, and saturated; and then there is trans fat which, essentially, is unsaturated fat gone bad—really bad. Polyunsaturated fat is considered to be the healthiest. So lets break it down, from best to worst:

POLYUNSATURATED FAT is "good fat." It is found in cold-water fish such as tuna, halibut, sardines, and salmon, as well as various types of plant oils including sunflower, safflower, soybean, and sesame seed. Polyunsaturated fat is in liquid form when at room temperature (think about a bottle of safflower oil). The reason why it is good for you is because it contains essential fatty acids (such as omega-3 and omega-6), which have been proven to promote health by reducing the risk of heart disease. It also helps maintain nerves and arteries, decreases skin problems, protects joints, and minimizes the risk of getting arthritis and some cancers.

MONOUNSATURATED FAT is also considered to be a good fat. It is found in olive oil, peanuts, avocado, canola oil, and some other nuts. It is usually in a liquid form when at room temperature (think of olive oil). Even the FDA backs this fat. In fact, olive oil is the only cooking oil to receive such FDA approval. So be sure to enjoy a daily dose of olive oil in your diet—2 tablespoons per day, to be exact, may reduce your risk of coronary heart disease. Monounsaturated fat helps maintain healthy levels of cholesterol by lowering LDL (bad cholesterol) and increasing levels of HDL (good cholesterol).

SATURATED FAT, on the other hand, is bad fat. Its only role in life is to be burned for energy. But when consumed in excess, with nowhere else to go, it glues itself to your hips and any other fat spots on your body. Americans notoriously eat too much saturated fat. Aside from making us a country filled with fat people, saturated fat also puts your liver on overdrive as it manufactures cholesterol, which clogs your arteries and causes heart attacks. Thankfully, saturated fat is easy to spot. It is usually solid at room temperature and often comes from animal fat. For example, red meat and butter are high in saturated fat. Ice cream, cheese, chocolate, and milk are also sources of saturated fat, as are coconut oil, palm oil, and palm kernel oil. Saturated fat is all-around bad. It contributes to heart disease and obesity. Avoid it.

Another type of fat that should be avoided is TRANS FAT. Trans fat is what happens when good fat turns bad. It is actually unsaturated fat that was hydrogenized, converting it from a liquid to a solid. The process of hydrogenation gives food a longer shelf life, but it also confuses the body into treating it similar to a saturated fat, but worse. Since it is not actually a saturated fat, food labels do not record it as such, allowing this bad fat to slip under the radar. Trans fats are in many common foods including cookies, crackers, fried foods, margarine, shortening, potato chips, french fries, and doughnuts. Similar to saturated fat, trans fat raises LDL (bad cholesterol) and increases your risk of heart disease. It is bad-bad-bad and should be cut out of your diet completely!

Rest

In order for your body to perform optimally each day, it needs time to repair itself and rest each night. While you get your beauty sleep, your body is working away to keep your immune system strong, pumping up your ability to respond to viruses and other harmful pollutants. Simultaneously, carbohydrates are being metabolized and fats broken down. You may feel relaxed, but as you sleep, your muscles are growing stronger, healing themselves from the day, particularly if you strength train. In fact, during waking hours while lifting weights, your muscles are actually weakening, slightly tearing with every curl. But it is those tears that fuse together as you sleep, gaining even more strength. Though your eyes may be closed, your mind is not completely at rest; it is filing away learned lessons of the day. Problems are being sorted out, answers to questions that you wracked your brain for hours earlier that afternoon are being found. Somehow, things seem to fall into place, without your conscious awareness, while you sleep. When you finally wake up, after a good night's sleep, your body is rested and ready to go, your mind is sharp and buzzing with information, and a few years seem to have reversed themselves from your face. But if you want your muscles, body, and mind to adequately heal, you need to give it enough time. Though everyone's rhythms and needs for sleep are slightly different, on average 8 hours of sleep is recommended each night.

Unfortunately, not everyone has the ability to lay their heads on a pillow and drift away for eight hours. Why? Our waking lives sometimes seem to get in the way. Late-night activities and early-morning appointments leach hours from our much-needed shut-eye. Once you finally get to sleep, a partner's snoring, a child's nightmare, or a neighbor's unnecessary noise can keep you wide-eyed and frustrated. But it isn't just time constraints, scheduling, and circumstance that steal our sleep. In fact, more than 70 million Americans suffer from a sleep disorder. You may be one of them. According to studies published in the medical journal *Sleep,* women, especially overweight women, are plagued with more sleep problems than men. If you are overweight and in the throws of menopause, yet you are not taking hormones, your chances of having trouble sleeping are even greater. Sleep disorders leave us tossing and turning for hours on end, or suddenly waking up in the middle of the night for seemingly no reason. Once you finally get to sleep, your alarm blares and it's time to attempt to peel your exhausted body from your bed and hit the shower! This consistent sleep deprivation is doing more harm than merely leaving you with dark circles under your eyes and a fuzzy head. In fact, when paired with driving, sleep deprivation can be hazardous or even fatal.

When you are tired, reaction times are significantly slowed and performance ability is reduced. Don't skip out on sleep, or you may experience one of the following repercussions:

- Decreasing your sleep time by just 1.5 hours for one night can decrease your alertness by as much as 32 percent.
- Your memory and ability to think clearly may be drastically impaired.
- Your relationships may suffer. Tossing and turning during the night will likely wake your partner, disrupting their sleep too. No one likes to be disturbed during a deep sleep. If mid-night disruptions are consistent, it may result in sleeping in different bedrooms, moodiness, and fights.
- Your quality of life may be affected, hindering your ability to participate in activities that require your uninterrupted attention, for example watching TV with your spouse, supporting your children by attending their dance and acting performances, going to the movies with friends. If you can't keep your eyes open, no one will want you as a movie partner.
- You might injure or kill yourself or someone else. This is when sleep deprivation gets really serious. According to estimates made by the National Highway Traffic Safety Administration, driving

while sleep deprived is the reason for at least 100,000 car crashes, 71,000 of which cause injury, and 1,550 of which cause death each year.

In addition to all of the above reasons why you should not neglect your precious hours of sleep, since this is a book about developing the perfect body, it is important to note that sleep deprivation can make you gain weight! *The Journal of Clinical Endocrinology & Metabolism,* November 2004, published a study suggesting that you are likely to eat more when sleep deprived. In fact, some sleepy study participants ate 1,000 calories more each day than the wide-eyed control group. Even if your stomach is actually full, you may feel hungry when you are sleepy. This confusion is caused by decreased leptin levels (a hormone thought to be the secret to obesity). Our levels of leptin notify the brain as to how hungry we are. When leptin levels are low, as is what happens when we don't get enough sleep, we feel hungrier. Getting enough sleep is considered to be crucial to a successful weight-loss plan, and to general health and well-being.

I am not just going to leave you there in the dumps, depressed about your inability to sleep and feeling like weight loss is impossible. There are things you can do to improve your sleep at night. Exercise is one of them. Stretching and working out for 1 hour in the morning has been proven to help relieve sleep problems. While exercise at any time of the day is great, in order to better your chances of having a good night of sleep, exercise in the morning has actually been scientifically proven to be more beneficial. In fact, when tested, women who already had sleep disorders were asked to exercise for 3.5 to 4 hours a week in the morning. By the end of the study, they had less trouble falling asleep. Women who exercised less than 3 hours per week in the morning did not notice a change in their ability to sleep. Women who exercised in the evening actually had more trouble falling asleep. It has been suggested that the reason for this sleep/exercise response is because exercise releases hormones and affects our body's temperature levels and our internal clocks. As the evening progresses, our body's temperature naturally starts to go down. Exercise has the opposite effect, as it increases our temperature. If evening exercise is the only time that you can fit into your schedule, don't worry, just be sure to allow your body 3 hours to cool down before hitting the sack and attempting to sleep.

Stress is often a reason why sleep is hindered. Exercise is one of the best stress relievers around. If your mind can't seem to shut off once the lights go out, there is a good chance that your sleep disorder is stress related. A regular fitness routine should minimize the way in which stress affects you, allowing you to deal with it more calmly and help ease your mind to sleep.

3

You are your body's architect. Build!

Body Basics — Body Awareness

We have successfully conquered outer space, yet we still struggle to understand inner space. To achieve this ultimate understanding, you've got to start with the basics.

More than a vessel for movement, allowing us to work and raise our kids, or a receptacle to fill with food, your body is an intricately assembled living thing with interconnected parts to support your life. Understanding the terminology and the how's and why's of particular muscles will help ensure that you get the most out of your workout. No, this is not about to turn into an in-depth physiology course; this is about the basics. You will soon be familiar enough to follow along with a trainer or instructor (in case you decide to go that route) when they try to impress you by rambling off body parts, with the soon-to-be incorrect assumption that you have no idea what they are talking about. It's kind of

41

like a car—mechanics are notorious for taking advantage of women, blathering off an extensive and expensive list of things your car needs in order to be sure that the engine doesn't drop out while you're driving. Please! You end up leaving the repair shop with $5,000 of unnecessary repairs. Knowledge is power, ladies. Take control of your body by understanding it.

> *Make the most of yourself, for that is all*
> *there is of you.*
> —EMERSON

Cardio Barre is fundamentally *body awareness,* focusing on isolating the smaller muscle groups, making you acutely aware of every inch of your body. This awareness assists in your understanding that if you move one muscle, another complementary muscle will, in turn, be triggered, allowing for a more efficient workout. Soon all of your movements will be initiated with awareness and carried through with intention. As you walk, you will be aware of the placement of your tailbone. If it is sticking out, rather than being tucked under, you will have the consciousness to make an adjustment, which will, in turn, relieve pressure from your lower back, allowing your spine to lengthen and your posture to improve. When you sit, you will feel the muscle fibers in your core activate, pulling up and in, creating an internal strength that assists your body as it repositions and changes its center of gravity. I am not saying that all you will be thinking about, all of the time, are the movements of your body, but those movements will constantly be in your unconscious mind, leaving room for a vibrantly lived conscious life.

To avoid injury and maximize your potential, when you work out on your own it is important that you are aware of your body's musculature and how to correctly work it. There are over 650 muscles in the body; you really need to know about 20 of them.

To begin to understand how your body works, let's start at the top.

Shoulders

Sexy shoulders look great with a Prada handbag hanging from them. But the bag won't be the only eye-catcher. Believe it or not, shapely shoulders can be even more appealing than a Chanel. Strong shoulders support the upper body. They are the force that drives your ability to lift more weight when working less developed muscle groups such as your chest and back.

Shoulder pads may be passé, but there is a reason they were sewn into every woman's suit coat and sweater for over a decade. I will let you in on a little Hollywood secret—broad shoulders make waistlines appear more slender. Need I say more? Developing your shoulder strength negates the need for extra padding and assists in the "hour glass" effect.

Back: Trapezius/Rhomboidens/Erector Spinae

"Back fat"—that taboo combination of words is the last thing anyone wants associated with them! Though you may not be able to see behind you without a three-way mirror, you have to address every angle. The back, one of the most neglected spots on the body when it comes to target toning, is just as important as your legs, arms, and abs. You may not see it, but believe me, everyone else does!

Yes, that bulging spot that loves to bubble over your bra strap is back fat! Unfortunately, fashion is consistently taking inches off once modest dress shirts. Sleeves are being torn off, necks cut low, and supposedly supportive fabric in the back are being minimized to a measly string! To follow fashion's trimming trend and feel comfortable in your new, though fewer, threads, it's time to concentrate on the, until now, ignored back!

Trapezius

Stave off neck and shoulder tension by toning your trapezius—the muscles in the upper center of your back. For those of you who consider a purse an extension of your home, and end up hauling the excessively heavy accessory until your shoulder aches, strong "traps" (trapezius) will allow you to lug the load with ease. They also accentuate the shape of your shoulders.

Rhomboideus

Rhomboids, the ever so subtle muscles that squeeze your shoulder blades together and eliminate the bra strap fat hangover that makes spaghetti straps risqué for some, must be flexed! More than making strapless tops your best friend, the rhomboids also assist in the perfecting of your posture.

Erector Spinae

One-third of the people in this country experience lower back problems. There's a good chance that you are one of them. Increasing strength in your erector spinae—the fancy term for the group of muscles that run from your tailbone up to the top of your spine—alleviates back pain and minimizes your chances of incurring injury. The added spine support also contributes to properly aligned posture, creating an illusion of extra inches added to your height.

Chest: Pectorals

Why are breast lifts and implants the accessory of the month? Because a perky bust is a heavily coveted commodity. Whether already accentuated or touting the beauty of your God-given gifts, there is always room for improvement . . . naturally! Just as you might exercise your calf muscles, you can actually accentuate your breasts by building the muscles below them.

Pectorals

Building the chest muscle under your breasts will accent and help lift them. Though you cannot make your breasts larger through exercise, you can make them appear firmer, lifted, and larger!

Arms: Triceps/Biceps/Forearms

Aside from your face and neck, your arms are the most exposed area of the body. So be sure they are always at their most shapely. Lifting low weight at high reps will create that lean, tone, long look that you like.

Triceps

Possibly more problematic than back fat is that unshakable underarm flap that makes "pointing over there" an insecurity-triggering gesture. Ahhh, the troublesome triceps! If you find that shaking a saltshaker shakes more than just salt, as your underarm fat bounces back and forth, you know what I am talking about. But, here's the good news. That flap isn't all fat! The bad news? From under use, your tricep muscle actually detaches from the bone and just hangs there, shaking away. Good news again? Cardio Barre can reattach and tighten that muscle right up!

Biceps

Biceps are for pulling and triceps are for pushing. More than beautiful extensions of your core, strong arms are functional in everyday life, making daily occurrences, like carrying your child and pushing the shopping cart, easier. Generally, men tend to have stronger upper bodies than women. That's why when you ask them to do the heavy lifting for you, it seems so easy for them. It can become easier for you too, making you stronger and more independent. But it's still fun to watch your man grunt as he puts the two gallon container of spring water on the dispenser, or carries the forty-pound bag of dog food from your car to the garage (not thinking about the fact that you carried it to the car from the store with the greatest of ease).

Abdominals: Rectus Abdominis/Internal and External Obliques

According to the current trends, pants are getting lower and tops are getting shorter, leaving little room to hide a flawed midsection. Yes, strong abs are sexy. And even a little pouch is cute. But, in addition to aesthetics, your abdominals support your back and help your posture. They also contribute to a strong lower back and in-line spine. But the honest truth about abs is that no matter how many ab exercises you do, you will not attain a flat tummy unless you remove the layer of fat around it. . . . Diet!Diet!Diet!

Rectus Abdominus

Your rectus abdominus is the long sheet of muscles that starts right below your chest and ends a few inches below your naval. This is one long muscle. It allows you to bend at the waist and works together with your lower back muscles to support and stabilize your torso while the rest of your body is moving. There is no such thing as "lower abs" or "upper abs." You may focus on specific portions of the rectus, but the entire muscle is worked during abdominal exercises.

Internal and External Obliques

Internal and external obliques run diagonally down the sides of your rectus abdominus. Your obliques are the enablers of the twisting motion. They also work with the other abdominal and back muscles to support your spine.

Butt and Hips: Gluteus Maximus/Hip Adductors/ Leg Adductors

A round, firm behind is something to be proud of. But no one wants too much "junk in the trunk." It's easy to work your butt off if you know the muscles to target.

Gluteus Maximus

The "glutes," also known as the butt, may be the largest muscles in the body, but they do not have to be the fattest! They cover the entire width of your derriere.

They help you climb stairs and hills, jump, and assist with sitting or standing. Those tight jeans and extra oomph short skirts do wonders, but a lifted butt doesn't have to be an illusion. The real test is: How does your butt look when getting out of the shower? Don't you want your partner to see it, in all of its glory, without the added lift from figure flattering clothes? If your buttocks are larger than you prefer, resistance training will make them firmer and more shapely, not bigger and bulkier. It's time to tighten that tush! Eliminate pantyline bulge, do away with butt dimples and burn those saddlebag pockets of fat. If you are one who sits all day on your rear end, then it would be a good idea to give those muscles the attention they deserve.

Hip Adductors

Otherwise known as the outer thigh or hip, hip adductors are muscles that help your leg slide out to the side, as if your were skating or stepping out of someone's way. These muscles work with your glutes to help turn your hips inwards. Strong adductors will help prevent hip injuries. These muscles are involved in almost every activity that involves the lower body. Strong adductors are important in maintaining a natural walking stride and preventing a lazy shuffle.

Leg Adductors

Leg adductors are also known as the inner thigh. They consist of several muscles that run along the inside of your hip to different points of the inner thigh. These muscles help you place one foot in front of the other. Strong inner thighs help you squeeze and stay on a horse or a motorcycle. Be careful of becoming obsessive and overworking your inner thighs, however, for they have a tendency to become inflamed.

Legs: Quadriceps/Hamstrings/Calves and Ankles/ Gastrocnemius and Soleus

Your legs bear a tremendous burden on a daily basis—you. It's time to trim, strengthen, and show them off.

Quadriceps

Your "quads" are the four muscles at the front of each thigh. They are responsible for straightening your knees. Keep strong quads to prevent knee problems. These muscles are also used for climbing, running, walking, hopping, skating, skiing, and jumping. Quads are typically very strong and developed. They have to be, since they are responsible for carrying you around! Imagine carrying 130, 170, 200, and up pounds all day long! Now you know what your legs are feeling. Since they are used to trekking around with a lot of weight, it is going to take more than a little cardio and a few leg lifts to really make an impact on your legs. Your quadriceps—the upper, frontal half of your legs—are already a massive muscle, before you even begin to work out.

Hamstrings

Your "hams" are the three muscles at the back of your thighs. They are responsible for bending the knee, as well as used in sitting and standing. Hamstring injuries are more common because they are usually much less developed than the stronger quads (their opposing force). Since your hams are so susceptible to pulls, make sure you warm them up properly before exercise or sporting activity. When bending over to touch your toes, if you feel tightness in the back of your thighs—those are your hamstrings.

Calves and Ankles

Ladies, I know the painful price you sometimes pay in order to strut around in your skyscraper high heels all night long. And, believe me, men appreciate it very much. Manolo Blahniks and high-heeled stilettos are undeniably sexy. But they will look even better with lean, toned calves and ankles to go with them, not to mention adding a bit of support to your stability-lacking sling-backs.

Gastrocnemius and Soleus

Your gastrocnemius and soleus (also known as your calves) are the large diamond muscles that give the back of your lower legs their shape. The calves allow you to stand up on your toes and spring off the floor when you jump with elation! Strong calves are good for dancing, jumping, running, or hopping. They help with long romantic walks or waiting in those hour-long lines! When they are shapely and strong, they are very sexy!

Terms and Proper Placement

Flat Back

Keep your body parallel to the floor, with your tummy pulled up, spine straight and head in line with your spine, like a table. Your torso is at a complete 90-degree angle and your legs are perpendicular to the floor. In order to maintain a flat back, your core is activated and your hamstrings are elongated. This is Flat Back.

Plié

Stand up straight. Now bend your knees, keep your tummy pulled in and maintain a straight spine—do not arch or contract your back. Lift your chest by pulling your shoulders back imagining that your shoulder blades are pinching your spine. This is where "opposition" comes in. As you bend your knees down, or "Plié," your torso lifts upward . . . lengthening and elongating.

Turnout

Make the shape of a V with your feet—heels together, toes apart. Turn your legs and hips outward, keeping your knees looking in the same direction as your toes. As you do a "Plié" or "Turnout," always keep your knees directly in line with your toes. In other words, if you were to drop a string directly down from your knees to the floor, it should land directly in front of your toes, not at all inside or outside. Do not force the Turnout. Work at your own natural flexibility. A 90-degree turnout is average, a 180-degree turnout is too much.

Torso Twist

The Torso Twist is an isolation. The motion is the twisting of your upper body from side to side without moving your hips, legs, or feet. Lead with your shoulders and rib cage and rotate from your waist. When one shoulder is in front of your body, the other should be in back.

Standing Posture

Yes, Standing Posture is simply standing, but the key is *how* you are standing. The average person slightly sticks out their neck, slumps their shoulders forward, and arches their lower back so that their butt protrudes. This is incorrect and will contribute to a misshapen spine. For Standing Posture, stand straight with your weight distributed evenly on both feet. Breathe in through your nose and out through your mouth, slightly expanding your belly as you inhale and pulling your stomach in and up (without raising your shoulders) as you exhale. Notice your stomach muscles contract, creating a hard protective shell over your internal organs as you exhale. This slims the waist. Pull your shoulders back, your chest out, and drop your tailbone by rotating your butt slightly under. Stand tall and confident.

It's All in the Details

It is possible that a position just won't feel quite right on your body. It oddly strains or you hear a pop. Remember that it is all in the details! Sometimes seemingly insignificant change can alter everything, and help click you into place mentally, physically, and emotionally. You need to get specific. Look at how an athlete prepares: a gymnast chalks up and makes sure her grip is perfect before leaping onto the balance beam. A boxer meticulously wraps his wrists and hands before entering the ring. These are not random obsessive-compulsive acts, but an integral part of their process, the means through which athletes center, focus, and bring themselves into the present . . . safely and without risk of injury. Do the same with your training, especially without a trainer present. Focus on all the subtleties: your posture, alignment, breath, and energy level. This is a thinking person's workout—THINK!

Goal Setting

Goals, both grand and immediate, help to keep you from working aimlessly. They will anchor your workout and help you chart progress. This means focused action and follow-through that supports what you are doing. The connection is pivotal and potent. Aim high, but be reasonable, and keep your eye on the goal. After 8 weeks of hard work and sweat, if you keep focused on your goals, you will obtain the slim physique that you so desperately want, you will better your life and find that you are smiling more, your eyes give off a glint, and your skin radiates with health and triumph! Not so bad for 8 weeks of work is it? If you really put your mind and your energy into achieving your goals, you will!

Set a Grand and an Immediate Intention

Why have you decided to pick up this book? What are you looking to achieve? Setting an intention, both a grand and an immediate intention, is one of the best ways to succeed because you have a designated goal, and you can devise a plan that will efficiently take you from point A to B, which eventually will bring you to Z. It is time to define your goals and clarify the differences between grand and immediate intentions.

Intentions can be set in a number of ways:

1. On the grand scale, why are you working out?
2. What do you wish to achieve?
3. You may have a grand intention, say, to lose 40 pounds, or be more flexible, maybe even both.
4. You may also have smaller, per-workout immediate intentions that support your grand intention.
5. The clearer you are about your goal or intention, the easier it is to gauge your success and evolution.

4

Women Need to Know

Menstrual Cycle and Fitness

"That time of the month" can be an emotional roller coaster for many women. Being surrounded by classes filled with women all day made me quickly realize how turbulent "that time of the month" can be. But you don't have to suffer though it. Exercise can actually help even out your PMS-related mood swings, minimize bloat, and decrease cramps. Look, I am not saying that if you are having one of those especially bad heavy days that you have to work out. Everyone deserves a break once in a while. But the fact is that women who keep up with their programs and regularly exercise, before and during their periods, have more energy, fewer cramps, and their tempers are tempered. As to your exercise performance when on your period, it shouldn't be negatively affected.

Actually, there are several studies suggesting that women, particularly endurance athletes, perform even better when menstruating! The reason could be because that annoying bloat, or water retention that puffs up your bodies,

Fit Tip

Relieve PMS symptoms by avoiding caffeine (coffee, tea, cola, and cocoa) and increasing exercise and relaxation (massage does wonders).

actually helps you to maintain better hydration. Of course, being bloated is never a reason to celebrate. Which is why you should exercise. When done in conjunction with a healthy, low-salt diet, exercise gets your juices flowing, including the extra water weight that you are carrying around. When working out, excess fluids are forced out of your tissues and into your blood stream, which are then excreted as sweat or urine, therefore de-bloating your body!

While I definitely suggest maintaining your exercise schedule throughout your cycle, if you dedicate only a few days to getting in shape, try to do it during the later menstrual phase. During that time, you have a high concentration of ovarian hormones, which promote the use of fat as energy. During aerobic activity, fat is a more efficient and clean-burning energy source. In translation—you will burn more fat and have more energy when exercising during the final phase of your menstrual cycle.

Keep in mind, though, that anything in excess can be bad. Yes, even exercise. Unfortunately, there is another side to the exercise/menstruation coin—and that is a loss of your period. Over-exercising and excess weight-loss can shift the normal hormonal balance and temporarily suspend your monthly cycle.

Pregnancy and Fitness

Pregnancy is no excuse for inactivity. In fact, unless directed by your doctor, it is the last thing you want to do. Approximately 42 percent of pregnant women in the United States exercise. How often and how hard vary according to the trimester (an increase in blood volume can cause women to get more tired faster), the presence of nausea, and general fatigue. Cardio Barre is the ideal exercise program for pregnancy because it follows all of the dos and don'ts of exercising while pregnant.

The Dos

- Do keep up a moderate exercise program unless otherwise advised by your doctor.
- Do focus on low- or no-impact exercises.
- Do concentrate on minimal-weight-bearing activities. Using light weights to increase upper strength is a good thing.
- Do wear breathable, loose-fitting, lightweight clothing to minimize an excess of heat and allow moisture to evaporate.
- Do stay hydrated throughout your workout.
- Do stretch after a workout.
- Do stick to a healthy diet and gain the recommended amount of weight, determined by your doctor.
- Do increase your heart rate to 50 to 60 percent of your maximal rate.

The Don'ts

- Don't exercise to the point of exhaustion. Take a break when you feel tired.
- Don't exercise lying on your back during your second and third trimesters.
- Don't exercise in hot, humid conditions.
- Don't do exercises that may disturb your abdomen or uterus.
- Don't do exercises that make you feel off balance or dizzy.
- Don't exercise on a completely empty stomach.
- Don't exercise if you have not gained enough weight.
- Don't exercise if you have preeclampsia, hypertension, heart disease, preterm labor, premature rupture of the membrane, or a weak cervix.
- Don't overdo it.

Regular physical activity can make your pregnancy, and even the birth, less uncomfortable by lifting your spirits, supporting your posture, relieving backaches, improving sleep, and minimizing weight gain. While you definitely want and need to gain weight (that is part of the fun of being pregnant), exercise helps counteract your excessive weight gain due to momentary lapses of judgment that lead you to eat an entire chicken instead of just the breast (yes, this really does happen—a lot).

Even if you never worked out regularly before pregnancy, it's never too late to start! After consulting with your doctor, you can ease into an exercise routine when pregnant. Just don't push yourself.

When your bun is finally baked and it is time to deliver, your continued dedication to exercise will pay off. Studies show that physically fit, active women enjoy easier labors, are less likely to need epidural analgesia, and require less medical intervention. Believe me, ladies, if 30 minutes of exercise, a few times a week, can take multiple hours and decimals of pain off your baby's birth, you will be so happy you did it.

Menopause and Fitness

Many women fear the onset of menopause because of the changes that occur, both physically and mentally. Other women can't wait for the day when they get to throw out their boxes of tampons and pads forever! Whatever your take on the change of life may be, be sure to keep your health in mind.

Menopause tends to take place in women between the ages of 48 and 52. It can occur as early as the late 30s or as late as the mid 50s. It is caused by a decrease in estrogen and other hormones produced by the woman's body. This causes a gradual reduction and finally a loss in a woman's period. As your hormones slowly diminish, your bones begin to become brittle and thin, which can lead to many other health problems. Exercise is very important during this time in order to preserve bone density and strength. But you can't just rely on your occasional evening strolls to maintain maximum health. Aerobic exercise and resistance training are both essential to keep your body in shape. Cardiovascular exercise (or aerobic exercise) keeps your heart strong and healthy, and keeps excess weight from piling on, while resistance training (or strength training) fortifies your bones and helps prevent osteoporosis.

The maintenance of your body is undeniably important, but another, sometimes hard-hit effect of menopause is your emotional state. PMS may be a thing of the past, but hot flashes could be in your future. A regular exercise routine has been proven beneficial when it comes to boosting your mood, warding off hot flashes, and improving sleep.

While working out the muscles in your body, don't forget to exercise those in your pelvis. The re-

Fit Tip

Hot flashes and other symptoms of menopause may be minimized by eating a diet rich in soybeans. A soy-rich diet may also reduce the risk of breast cancer. Soy and other legumes (beans, yams, etc.) contain phytoestrogens, compounds that may mimic estrogen–replacement therapy for menopausal symptoms.

duction in hormones can also reduce your sex drive. Kegel exercises help increase blood flow and strengthen the pelvic muscles—PC (pubococcygeus) muscles, therefore increasing sexual arousal pleasure. Daily Kegel exercises also help maintain bladder control, preventing incontinence. Kegel exercises can be done anywhere—in the car, watching TV, lying in bed—without anyone noticing. Your PC muscle is what you use to stop the flow of urine while going to the bathroom. When your bladder is empty, practice squeezing that muscle as if you were attempting to stop the flow of urine. Squeeze for 3 seconds. Then release. Repeat several times until your muscles begin to feel tired. You can also try longer holds as well as several short flutters. Suddenly, boring meetings and being stuck in traffic isn't so bad!

More than whittling your middle and saving your sex life, exercise can help maintain the strength of your heart. As a woman's heart ages, cholesterol buildup can cause the artery walls to thicken, triggering heart disease and increasing the risk of stroke. According to the *Journal of the American College of Cardiology,* exercise can significantly lessen the effect, slowing the progression of disease. In general, women have a lower risk of heart disease than men. But, as women near menopause, their risk increases, equaling, and sometimes surpassing that of men.

Depression may also be a symptom of menopause, a problem that exercise can help manage. Endorphins (sometimes referred to as "happy hormones") released in the brain during exercise can help improve your mood and alleviate symptoms of stress.

Exercise helps manage menopause by:

- Helps prevent weight gain, especially around the stomach
- Minimizes your risk of osteoporosis by maintaining bone mass and strength
- Improves your mood and reduces mood swings
- Lowers your risk of heart disease and high blood pressure
- Sustains sexual functioning
- Can reduce hot flashes
- Improves sleep

Understanding Fat and Cellulite

Yes, I said it, "cellulite"! It is the dreaded word that we all try to stay as far away from as possible. Almost hard to let it roll off your tongue isn't it? If you have this skin condition, you are not alone. Approximately 85 percent of women are affected by it. Even skinny people have cellulite. It's just that they have less surface area to show it off. Yes, contrary to popular belief, the lumpy, dimply, "orange peel" appearance of cellulite occurs on all shapes and sizes—thin, average, and overweight—not just on obese bodies. *Change* is actually the impetus for cellulite. Changes in blood flow, lymphatic drainage, fat, connective tissue, hormone balance, and lifestyle all contribute to the unsightly sacks of fat. Unfortunately the physiological changes that occur due to the existence of cellulite can worsen over time, thanks to poor lifestyle choices including lack of exercise, poor diet, insufficient water consumption, and then there is the inevitable—aging.

As we age, our bodies naturally lose tone as muscle and skin turns to flab. Our connective tissues have a similar response to added years. Their thickness and resiliency slacken, making cellulite more visible. The rippled dimples are most often found on the hips, buttocks, and legs. Though labeled as fat, cellulite is actually a combination of fat, water, and "toxic wastes" that the body has collected in the form of deposits, instead of eliminating, as it should. It is the result of poor circulation, weak connective tissue, hormonal imbalance, fluid retention, and, most often, genes (not jeans that you wear, but inherited genes—thanks Mom and Dad!). As you have probably noticed, fat cells on the lower body are better at hanging on for dear life than fat cells on the upper body—translation: you probably have more fat on the lower half of your body than on the upper half. No, it is not just you. Fat cells on your butt, thighs, and legs are 6 times stronger, making them more likely to stick and be stored. The frustrating outcome of such resiliency is that it is much more of a challenge to get rid of lower body fat than it is to get rid of upper body fat. Let me break it down for you.

Connective Tissue

Beneath the skin lies a layer of collagen fibers and fatty cells that support the organs and fill any open spaces between them. They also form the tendons and ligaments. Connective tissues run up and down, perpendicularly, at a 90-degree angle from the muscles, through the fat, and connect to the undersurface of the skin. This configuration allows for lumps, bulges, and wrinkles to misshape the skin (the connective fibers in men crisscross at a 45-degree angle, avoiding the skin creasing). When the connective issue is weak, it allows fat to penetrate it, pushing through and causing fat pockets known as cellulite. Strong tissue prevents the fat from pushing through and revealing itself.

Fluid Retention

Did you ever notice how your favorite pair of jeans will fit one day and be snug the next? No, you didn't suddenly gain 5 pounds, you are probably just retaining too many fluids. Salt and PMS are two of many causes for bloat, or water retention. Aside from being uncomfortable and giving you the unnecessary scare that you gained a lot of weight overnight, fluid retention can also cause swelling in the connective tissues, weakening them and potentially opening the door for fat to enter.

Hormonal Imbalance

Cellulite tends to develop during times of hormonal shifting, such as puberty, when taking birth control pills, during times of PMS, pregnancy, and menopause. Once puberty hits, the body changes for good thanks to the release of estrogen. Though it certainly has its benefits, such as giving you the ability to bear children, few benefits lack drawbacks. Estrogen is no exception. In preparation for childbearing, estrogen assists in the storage of fat in the hips, thighs, and butt. It also makes that fat sticky so that it can easily bunch together. The naturally occurring female hormone can also weaken connective tissue (is everything working against you?). The presence of estrogen softens the tissue around the womb to make childbirth possible, while also softening the thighs. Women with higher levels of estrogen may have an easier childbirth, but will likely have more cellulite.

Poor Circulation

Poor circulation can also cause swelling in the connective tissue. When your fluids are having trouble flowing, they tend to accumulate in certain areas before moving through. This accumulation can stretch the connective tissue, weakening its resiliency and allowing more of the fat to surface.

Inheritance

Being in the inheritance business can be a very good thing if what you are inheriting is money, a business, or great skin. But come on, Mom. Did you have to give me the cellulite? Yes, if your mom has it, you likely will too. If you have thin skin, which you can also thank Mom for, your cellulite will be even easier to see! If your connective tissue is loosely woven, guess what, fat will find it much easier to rear its ugly head through the fibers and make your skin bulge. If you are plagued with poor blood or lymphatic circulation, toxins will have a harder time moving through and out of your system, causing the caustic accumulation of waste—hello cellulite!

Lifestyle

Your lifestyle has a lot to do with the state of your health and your body. Emotional stress has been known to weaken connective tissue, therefore contributing to the accumulation of fat in the form of cellulite. It seems like every day there is yet another study that comes out underscoring the damage that stress does to our bodies. We need to find a way to de-stress and learn to relax more. Exercise is an excellent mode to de-stress. I can't talk enough about the benefits of exercise. So move that body of yours!

To make matters worse, the clumpy, fatty substance is often resilient to "cellulite reducing" creams and other quick-fix treatments. If you want to rid your skin of the sticky situation, one of the only treatment options that can cure you of cellulite is exercise. Exercise can specifically target the fat that subsists under loose skin, firming up the muscle and making it appear tight and smooth, while enhancing circulation and eliminating waste.

Has this been a scary enough section for you? My point? I will show you how exercise and nutrition will help in hormonal balance, better circulation, less stress, and stronger connective tissue. It will also help you lose fat and the monster . . . "Cellulite!"

You can best see cellulite when you are standing on your feet. To spot your cellulite, stand naked with your back to a mirror and look over your shoulder at your backside. If you see dimpled wrinkles and depressions, it's time to start working out to fight that stubborn fat. Use the Nurnberger-Muller Scale (below) to figure out the severity of your cellulite based on a four-stage scale, Stage 0 being normal skin and Stage 3, severe cellulite.

Nurnberger–Muller Scale

Stage 0

When you stand on your feet or lie on your back, there is no visible dimpling. Pinching a few inches of skin between your fingers (the "pinch test") makes your skin fold or crease, but not dimple like cottage cheese.

Stage 1

When you stand on your feet or lie on your back, there is no visible dimpling; but the pinch test tells a different story, revealing a few dimples and a cottage cheese appearance.

Stage 2

When you stand on your feet dimpling naturally appears, but when you lie on your back there is no visible dimpling.

Stage 3

When you stand on your feet or lie on your back, dimpling naturally appears.

To help combat cellulite there are several things you can do, including:

- Up your water intake to at least 8 glasses of water per day.
- Minimize coffee, tea, and alcohol consumption.
- If you can't let go of your morning cup of joe or evening glass of wine, drink 2 glasses of water for every serving of coffee, tea, or alcohol.
- Do Cardio Barre.
- Reduce your intake of saturated fat and carbohydrates and increase the amount of fruit, vegetables, and whole grains in your diet.

5

Prepare—A New Beginning

I know that new beginnings can be frightening, especially when you have failed time and time again. But standing in the way of your success due to a fear of failure is going to get you nowhere fast. Do not be afraid of starting this new beginning, of taking this journey to health, weight loss, and happiness. Dedicate one solid week to your success, and you have already succeeded. Because you are doing this program at home, there isn't a huge class of seasoned Cardio Barre-ites to intimidate you. The only person you are competing with is yourself. Prove to yourself that you can do this. Allow yourself to experience all of the pleasures and happiness that you have dreamt about. Cardio Barre is more than a program that sculpts a stronger body, it creates a stronger mind, body, and spirit. Use this time that you dedicate to yourself each day as a source of power. As your perfect body begins to take shape, your mind will follow; and, soon, your life will be have some of the perfection that you've always wanted. Let yourself have that happiness. You deserve it.

Medical Evaluation

You should always get a physical from your doctor before starting a new workout program. Your doctor will check things like your blood pressure, cholesterol, and blood sugar readings, basically examining your health history. Your doctor will give you the okay to begin as well as the particulars of the dos and don'ts of the exercise and diet appropriate for you.

Self-assessment

If I were meeting with you in person for the first time, I would make an assessment of your strengths and weaknesses in order to determine your fitness level and establish reasonable goals. Part of my evaluation would be from my observance of your body, the way you move, and your overall attitude. I would also ask you a series of questions and use your responses to gauge your aptitude. Since I am here and you are there, I am depending on you to judge yourself honestly through these tests. This is for your benefit, and it is a good way to get started. Be honest with yourself. There is no judgment.

Fitness Evaluation

The point of the fitness evaluation is to determine and be aware of your physical strengths and weaknesses. This awareness will help dictate what you need to work on, what areas of the body need more attention, or not as much. Keep in mind that this evaluation is a starting point from which you can only go up, get better, grow stronger! It is not meant to be frustrating or discouraging. If you don't do as well as you might have expected, don't worry, you are in the majority. There are plenty of people, even celebrities and models, whose initial fitness evaluations are less than impressive. But sometimes it is honesty and reality that works as your best motivator to make change. You are not required to be in perfect shape already. That's why you are starting this new workout plan. Use the fitness evaluation and allow it to empower you to achieve greatness!

Physical Fitness Tests

Below are standard self-assessment tests that have been used by trainers, doctors, and fitness experts to determine the physical strength of their clients. They were created for healthy adults with no existing disabilities that might restrict exercise. Remember, this is not a competition with anyone but yourself. Please do not push yourself beyond your limits. Use common sense. If you have been physically inactive or you are over the age of 40, please consult your physician before beginning any exercise program. Have fun!

Push-Up/Arm Strength

Do as many push-ups as you can.

Do "standard" push-ups (hands and toes touching the floor) or "bent-knee" push-ups (hands and knees are on the floor, lower legs and feet are bent up to the ceiling in a V). Keep your back and neck straight and aligned. Place your hands directly under your shoulders. Bend your elbows and lower your body down until your arms are bent to 90 degrees. You don't want to go lower than that. Be sure to keep your body straight as a board, making sure not to raise your butt higher than the rest of your body. Check your number with the chart.

AGE	17–19	20–29	30–39	40–49	50–59	60–65
EXCELLENT	more than 35	more than 36	more than 37	more than 31	more than 25	more than 23
GOOD	27–35	30–36	30–37	25–31	21–25	19–23
ABOVE AVERAGE	21–27	23–29	22–30	18–24	15–20	13–18
AVERAGE	11–20	12–22	10–21	8–17	7–14	5–12
BELOW AVERAGE	6–10	7–11	5–9	4–7	3–6	2–4
POOR	2–5	2–6	1–4	1–3	1–2	1
VERY POOR	0–1	0–1	0	0	0	0

Squat Test/Leg Strength

Use a chair that allows you to bend your knees at a 90-degree angle. Stand in front of the chair, with your back to the chair and your feet shoulder-width apart. You do not need to hold on to anything. You will maintain a center of balance. Bend your knees, stick your butt out, and squat down in a sitting position until you lightly touch the seat with your butt, then stand back up. Repeat until your legs are fatigued. Check your number with the chart.

AGE	18–25	26–35	36–45	46–55	56–65	65+
EXCELLENT	more than 43	more than 39	more than 33	more than 27	more than 24	more than 23
GOOD	37–43	33–39	27–33	22–27	18–24	17–23
ABOVE AVERAGE	33–36	29–32	23–26	18–21	13–17	14–16
AVERAGE	29–32	25–28	19–22	14–17	10–12	11–13
BELOW AVERAGE	25–28	21–24	15–18	10–13	7–9	5–10
POOR	18–24	13–20	7–14	5–9	3–6	2–4
VERY POOR	0–18	0–20	0–7	0–5	0–3	0–2

Abdominal Muscle Strength

Lie flat on your back. Extend your arms straight against your sides. To mark your finger location, place a strip of tape at the end of your fingertips. Place another strip 3 inches beyond the first strip (toward your toes). Sit up only slightly, keeping your lower back on the floor and curling your rib cage toward your pelvis. Your fingers should move only from the first strip of tape to the next. Relax back down. Repeat until you are unable to lift into a crunch even once more. How many times could you sit up? An excellent score for women is 50 repetitions.

AGE	Under 35	36–45	Over 45
EXCELLENT	50	40	30
GOOD	40	25	15
AVERAGE	25	15	10
POOR	10	6	4

Flexibilty

CAUTION: Perform this test gently and without sudden sharp movements. If you feel any pain, stop immediately. It is a good idea to warm up before you begin, in order to avoid injury.

Sit on the floor with your legs straight out in front of you with your feet about 10-inches apart. Place a yardstick vertically between your legs, with your heels aligned with the 15-inch mark on the stick (and the number getting higher as the stick continues past your toes). Tape the yardstick to the floor so that it doesn't move. Place one hand on top of the other in front of you. Stretch your torso forward, sliding your fingers along the yardstick until you have reached as far as you can. Write down (to the nearest inch) the number that you were able to reach. Repeat 3 times and use the highest number as your final score.

AGE	20–29	30–39	40–49	50–59	60+
HIGH	22 and up	21 and up	20 and up	19 and up	18 and up
AVERAGE	16–21	15–20	14–19	13–18	12–17
BELOW AVERAGE	13–15	12–14	11–13	10–12	9–11
LOW	12 or less	11 or less	10 or less	9 or less	8 or less

Cardiovascular Endurance

In order to perform this test, you will need to use a sturdy step or a stair. Use a step or chair that is not more than one foot off the ground. Step up onto the step with one foot, then up with the other. Then take one foot down back to the floor, followed by the other. Continue switching feet at a steady pace for 3 minutes.

Immediately after you are finished, check your pulse for 1 minute. Compare your pulse with the chart.

AGE	18–25	26–35	36–45	46–55	56–65	65+
EXCELLENT	under 85	under 88	under 90	under 94	under 95	under 90
GOOD	85–98	88–89	90–102	94–104	95–104	90–102
ABOVE AVERAGE	99–108	100–111	103–110	105–115	105–112	103–115
AVERAGE	109–117	112–119	111–118	116–120	113–118	116–122
BELOW AVERAGE	118–126	120–126	119–128	121–129	119–128	123–128
POOR	127–140	127–138	129–140	127–135	129–139	129–134
VERY POOR	over 128	over 138	over 140	over 135	over 139	over 134

Diet Evaluation

Nutrition is an essential element to a well-rounded wellness plan. Some experts say that diet is 50 percent of the battle. Nutritional deficiencies can result in grave health problems—including the increased risk of developing cardiovascular disease, cancer, and diabetes—many of which can be reduced by making good food choices. More than minimizing your chances of developing such diseases, eating healthfully can improve your energy level, mood, and enhance your immune system. Good nutrition involves eating enough (but not too much), having regular meals, and choosing the right foods in order to get all of your essential nutrients, such as vitamins, minerals, and protein that your body needs to stay healthy. Later on I will teach you to make healthier choices and improve on each of the topics addressed below.

A few diet questions to consider now are:

Am I conscious of portion control?	YES or NO
Do I drink plenty of water daily?	YES or NO
Do I check food labels?	YES or NO
Do I plan and prepare my meals in advance?	YES or NO
Do I make healthy substitutions?	YES or NO
Do I aim for high fiber and low fat?	YES or NO
Do I eat enough fruits and vegetables?	YES or NO
Do I eat a minimal amount of sugar?	YES or NO
Do I choose lean meats or proteins?	YES or NO

You should have answered yes for most, if not all, of the above questions. If you answered no to any of them, those are a few of the nutritional issues that you may need to improve on.

Mental Evaluation

In many instances, your mental health begins with your physical health. Studies suggest that physical activity, balanced nutrition, rest, and avoiding the abuse of alcohol and drugs greatly reduces your risk of mental illness.

Healthy eating habits are essential for your brain to function efficiently. In fact, your brain uses up to 20 percent of the energy produced by your body. Therefore, diet has a direct correlation with brain ability and activity. If you indulge in a diet that lacks fundamental nutrients that would keep your brain powered up to perfection, you are potentially lowering your learning ability, impairing your memory, depleting your energy, minimizing your patience and tolerance levels, and increasing sensitivity to stressors. And that is just the beginning of the detrimental devastation that you can wreak on your mind, let alone your body.

The Stress Test

Stress is the "fuel" that allows you to tap into your energy reserves in response to an unusual situation or to help you beyond the norm. Unfortunately, we live in a highly stressful society, in which we all too often say, "I am so stressed." Stress, in that context, is a negative. When we are constantly in a state of stress, we are taxing our bodies and minds, depleting our energy stores, and throwing our systems into a frenzy. It's like the boy who cried wolf. If you are constantly calling upon support from your body systems to expend extra energy to help in "unusually high stress" situations all of the time, you are dramatically decreasing your body's potential to come to your defense. People respond differently to stress, but if kept under control, stress can actually be used in a positive manner. Some people say that they "thrive" on stress. In other words, when under pressure they actually excel instead of falter. In order to replenish energy stores, remember that balance is key.

Factors that may make you prone to stress:

- *Unhealthy lifestyle habits* such as poor nutrition, physical inactivity, lack of sleep, and substance abuse.
- *Personality traits,* including: insecurity, a need to be in constant control of your surroundings, obsessive tendencies, a relentless desire for perfection, or a low tolerance for change. *Social skills,* such as lack of social life, inability to manage conflict, and poor support circle also contribute to an increased risk of stress.
- *Physical inactivity.* A physically active lifestyle improves your stress tolerance. When you exercise, your body releases chemicals that improve your mood. This explains the euphoric feeling, sometimes referred to as "runner's high," that you may feel up to

48 hours after a workout session. Being physically active also improves self-confidence and acts as a positive outlet for the release of anxiety, stress, and frustration. It can improve your sleep patterns and directly impact your mental and physical health. Exercise can even improve your social life.

- *Drug or alcohol abuse.* When feeling stressed many people turn to alcohol or drugs to "take the edge off," when, in actuality, more damage than good is being done. Alcohol and drugs are an unhealthy outlet for stress release. Though you may momentarily feel a reprieve from an anxious mind or frayed nerves, your body is under a tremendous amount of stress as it attempts to avoid and repair itself from the damage being done by the substances. Bottom line: Cut out drugs completely. Minimize your use of alcohol, or avoid it altogether.

Do you regularly experience any of the following signs of stress?

PHYSICAL SIGNS

Loss of appetite	YES or NO
Disrupted sleep	YES or NO
Headaches	YES or NO
Fatigue	YES or NO
Muscle spasms	YES or NO
Skin rashes	YES or NO
Tooth grinding	YES or NO
Back pain	YES or NO
Repetitive colds or flu	YES or NO

MENTAL SIGNS

Memory loss	YES or NO
Decreased motivation	YES or NO
Difficulty in decision making or concentrating	YES or NO

BEHAVIORAL CHANGES

Irritability	YES or NO
Trouble controlling temper	YES or NO
Loss of sexual desire	YES or NO
Antisocial behavior	YES or NO
Increased substance abuse	YES or NO

Stress may lead to low self-respect, depression, or violence. It can also increase the risk of cardiovascular disease or other diseases.

Tips for Stress Relief

Eat well.

Maintain a physically active lifestyle.

Get plenty of sleep.

Understand your stressors and try to correct them by starting new healthy patterns.

Confide in someone you trust.

Be less demanding on yourself and others.

Laugh at your mistakes.

Avoid overspending.

Learn to resolve conflicts in a positive way.

Know your limits and learn to say "no."

Change your attitude.

Don't hesitate to seek professional help.

Limit or cut out alcohol use.

What You Need

Hardware

You don't have to endure the aggravation of the gym in order to work out. You can actually never leave your house, and, with minimal equipment, still get a full-body, heart-pounding, sweat-dripping workout!

Thankfully, this is a fact that many Americans are finally becoming privy to. According to the Sporting Goods Manufacturers Association (SGMA), we spent approximately $4.2 billion on at-home exercise equipment in 2003, triple the $1.3 billion spent in 1990. Considering the billions of dollars spent on exercise, we are clearly on the right track. But exercise doesn't have to be so costly. In fact, you don't even need one electricity-powered, space-hogging machine. All you need is a sturdy, hip-high surface and a couple of weights.

Barre

In this book and in my classes we use a ballet barre. If you want to use the portable Cardio Barre, as in the pictures throughout the book, you can order it online at cardiobarre.com. If not, use a sofa, chair, or counter top. The height should be approximately hip level or slightly higher. Regardless of what you choose, be sure to find something stable that can support your weight.

Weights

You will also need a pair of 1- or 2-pound free weights, which can be purchased at any sporting goods store. If one is not easily accessible, and you want to get started right away, you can find objects of equal weight and size in your kitchen! Use two cans of soup, or bottles of water in place of the pair of weights.

Mat or Carpeted Floor

In addition to barre work, we incorporate floor work—that's dance-speak for exercises done on the floor. It is best to use a mat during floor work in order to protect your back from pain or injury. A carpeted floor may be enough padding. Lie on your back and feel for yourself. If your spine uncomfortably pushes into the ground, you need more padding. But don't go to extremes; a bed is too soft. It gives too much and can minimize the effectiveness of your exercises. You may think I am acting like the Princess and the Pea, but there are reasons for these specifications, you will see. I just don't want to waste any of your valuable time. You deserve to get the absolute most out of every second that you are working out.

Music

Because we will be doing cardio at the same time as the resistance work, we don't take any breaks, rest periods, or breathers (except when switching from one section to the next, but that counts more as a pause than a break). In fact, during the entire duration of your workout, you are moving your body. Music is a great motivator to keep moving. But not just any music—avoid slow, relaxing tunes, which are more apt to put you to sleep than urge you to jump up and shake your bon-bon. High-energy, pumping, rhythmic music is best. I am talking about the kind of music that naturally makes your hips sway, toes tap, and head nod. So long as it is fast, I have no preference as to the music style—rock, rap, rave, disco, eighties, or swing, doesn't matter to me, as long as it gets your body moving! Music makes the workout more fun and helps to redirect your attention from any uncomfortable exercises and place your mind on the music, pushing your body to work just a little bit harder!

Water

You will be losing a substantial amount of water during this workout, both through your mouth and through your pores. With each exhale a finite amount of water escapes from your system (think about when you breathe onto a mirror and you leave a mist on the glass—that is water). As you begin to breathe more deeply, exhaling more frequently, you lose even more water. Sweating secretes more than just toxins from your pores: there is a tremendous amount of water that you may not even be aware of since much of it evaporates into the air the second it reaches the surface of your skin. It is essential that you replenish your system by drinking a lot of water.

Clothing

Dress the part! Fitness clothing can actually act as motivation, pushing you to work out and look your best. Just as tennis necessitates the little white tennis skirt and white tennis shoes; ice skating calls for white skates and something warm on top; basket-

> **Fit Tip**
>
> Drink Water! Drinking more water and fewer liquid calories will suppress your hunger, lower your calorie intake, cleanse your body, and give you more energy.

ball, soccer, baseball, and every other sport calls for a certain outfit that makes you look *and* feel the part; so does a gym workout. Of course, it is not mandatory that you model designer threads that are so expensive that you actually fear sweating in them and getting them dirty—*gasp!* That would defeat the purpose. But when you decide to start a new exercise program, get a new pair of shoes and comfortable sweats to go with it. After all, you are preparing to begin a new, successful journey. So dedicate yourself to this new you by beginning anew, starting with your outfit. Fitness clothing is designed to be comfortable, flexible, and body conscious. You should stay away from anything too baggy that will hinder your movement and hide your beautiful body. Yes, your body is beautiful, even if you think you have a few pounds to lose. Tighter fitting clothes will allow you to see your body and check out your muscles in the mirror while being sure that you maintain alignment and proper placement.

While an outfit that is baggy enough that you can move, but not so baggy that it completely hides your body, is important, it is also important that you find clothes that flatter your body. Considering that you are going to be losing weight, quite possibly quickly, you don't want to spend everything you have on one perfect outfit—be prepared to buy a couple during this journey. But each additional outfit will be a gift to yourself, celebrating your accomplishments and allowing you to show off your new-found figure that was hiding under all that fat.

Once you have shed a few sizes, reward yourself with a great new outfit that emphasizes your chiseled-down figure. Try to go just a little tighter than you might normally opt for. But don't just shop for exercise clothes, splurge on a new pair of jeans. There is nothing more exhilarating than fitting into your "thin" jeans for the first time in five years or trying on a pair of jeans two sizes smaller than you originally were and having them fit—perfectly! As your body tightens, your face will likely change in shape too. A new hairdo that highlights your cheek bones can go a long way in the unveiling of the new you.

After your first trip to the mall, carrying an armful of clothes that are too big into the dressing room, you might, just for a second, wish you had your old body back. Why? Because nothing fits! It might not be that the clothes are just too big, but you might find that they are tight on your hips but loose on your stomach, or tight on your chest, but loose on your arms. Don't let this aggravation overcome you and make you turn to baggy sweatpants (which are only asking for you to fill them up again). It isn't your body that you should blame, but the clothing industry! Sizes are often designed from a "basic" shape. Unfortunately, the "basic" shape of Americans has been gradually evolving, and the clothing industry is slow to catch up. The standard American shape, according to the clothing industry, is the hourglass shape. The standard shape of women today is actually pear-shaped, with hips wider than shoulders. It is hard to stuff a pear into an hourglass without certain parts getting smashed and other parts feeling too roomy. If you feel like you are shoving a square into a circle when you are trying on clothes, you are not alone. In fact, you are part of the majority.

Have you ever tried something on that you swore looked bigger than the tag said, and, just because you fit into the one that is two sizes smaller than you normally are, you bought it (even though you really didn't love it)? That is another classic problem with clothing today—"vanity sizing." In order to make women feel better about the "size" of their clothing, some companies label a size 8 a size 4 or a size 12 an 8. That is the reason that you try on one pair of jeans and they fit like a glove, and another pair of jeans in the same size but a different designer and you feel like you are swimming in them. The outcome can be a very frustrating shopping experience. For example, a Spiegel catalog listed a 1X shirt as equal to a size 14–16, while Lane Bryant said that their 1X was the equivalent of a size 22–24. Just because the tag says it's a 4, 6, 8, 10, 12,

14, etc., and so are you, doesn't mean that it will fit you. If you find a line of clothing that fits well, stick with it.

The "Tester Skirt"

You have likely never heard of a "tester skirt" before, and that's okay. Laurel came up with this brilliant method of measuring her weight loss and gain by designating one specific skirt as her "tester skirt." A "tester skirt" is a skirt that is actually sizeless. In Laurel's case, it was her favorite skirt from college that she had taken-in in order to perfectly fit her figure. Since it had been altered, it lost the stigma of any particular size—it simply represents her shape. Laurel no longer wears this skirt out; its sole function is to measure her size loss and gain (which negates the need to wash the skirt and therefore accidentally shrink it). Instead of being a slave to the scale, Laurel tries on her "tester skirt" once a month and varies her workout and food program according to the skirt's fit. If you have a skirt that represents your "ideal" size, designate it as your "tester skirt" and toss your scale!

What to Expect

Start Slowly!

There is no need to jump into a full-on exercise program 5 days a week for an hour each day immediately. You are just asking to burn out, and fast. The key to beginning and maintaining a successful exercise routine that will last a lifetime and become truly a regular routine in your life, is by starting at a pace that you can dedicate yourself to and keep up with. Once you are comfortable in a routine, gradually add on to it, making sure to constantly challenge your body and mind. At the beginning, when you are attempting to set aside exercise time in an already busy schedule, if you think that you have to carve out 60 minutes, you are less likely to "find the time," whereas 30 minutes may seem more manageable at first, and you are more likely to find that time to dedicate to yourself. Once you can successfully schedule 30 minutes, 10 more minutes won't seem like such a stretch. After a few weeks at 40 minutes, another 10 minutes, making it 50 minutes, will still be realistic. Finally, after adjusting to 50 minutes, squeezing in another 10 minutes, therefore dedicating a full hour to your workout, will be very doable. Sometimes it is just about how you view things.

Similarly, if you work out so hard the first day that you can't walk for an entire week, you will probably be less inclined to take the time to exercise again anytime soon for fear that you will, again, be unable to walk for yet another week. Don't set yourself up for failure and discouragement. Don't injure yourself unnecessarily. Give your muscles a chance to readjust to the newly found stress of exercise so that your body can prepare itself to build muscle properly. Take it slow. Let your body and your schedule adjust to this new routine that you are incorporating into your lifestyle, which will soon become a lifestyle in itself. Take baby steps and grow gradually. Your body is like a car on a cold morning. It needs to gradually warm up before it can drive at top speeds without damaging the engine. You are the engine . . . warm it up.

Together, we will work consistently and patiently, keeping your goals in sight. After a few weeks, your body will be ready for a tougher routine and we will intensify your workout. Remember, this is about you and your success. I am here to help you obtain it . . . and you will, if you trust me.

Emotional Challenge

Changing your life can be more than physically exhausting, it can be emotionally draining too. Escaping unhealthy behavioral patterns, looking for a new comfort that doesn't involve food, and rewiring your exercise mentality can trigger the release of emotional baggage that needs to be sifted through and discarded in order to move forward. If you want the physical pounds to come off, you first have to lose the emotional pounds that sometimes weigh you down even more than your actual weight. You have to work at changing the way you eat, move, and think. You need to make a commitment to improve your life in all areas by tapping into resources of motivation and confidence that you never knew existed. You will learn to control your emotions, allowing you to make healthier choices, embracing this lifestyle change as a positive. This book is for more than shaping your perfect body (though that is a given). It is about you taking control of your life and attaining everything you want.

It's about more than the bike.

—LANCE ARMSTRONG

Feed Your Body

Before we even open the refrigerator and address the food options that will shape your new eating plan, it is important that we dive into the topic of water.

Water

Water is one of your body's most important elements. It makes up over half of your body (yes, water weight really is an excuse), 75 percent of which is your muscle tissue. It makes up 25 percent of your fatty tissue and is present within each cell, acting as transportation for vital nutrients and the dumping of waste. It is so essential that it is impossible to live more than a week without replenishing it. Why is it so important? Water regulates your body's temperature, helps maintain your internal organs, cushions and protects your vital organs, supports your digestive system, and sustains your energy. It is indispensable to all internal organs, which is why it is so important that we constantly replenish it throughout the day. Even when not exercising we are losing water through our breath, our pores, our sweat glands, and when exercising it dissipates at a much faster rate. It is your body's self-regulating cooling system, releasing heat in the form of sweat. Depending on the intensity of exertion (which should be pretty high with my exercise program) and the temperature of the air, you can lose about a quart of water! That's one wet shirt! The danger of so much water loss, without replenishing it, is dehydration. When you are dehydrated, your body loses its ability to cool itself, which may lead to heat exhaustion. In addition to temperature regulation, without sufficient water, your energy level will drop and your muscle function will suffer, causing cramps and fatigue. If you feel thirsty, you are already dehydrated. Drink water throughout the day to be safe. This is not to scare you away from exercising; it is to scare you into drinking water! When exercising, it is important to drink before, during, and after a workout. The more hydrated you are, the more energy you will have, the better your body will function for a longer period of time, the more calories you will burn, the more fat you will lose, and the sooner you will be thinner!

The Basics of Water and Your Workout

- To allow the assimilation of water into your body and benefit from its effects, drink 1 to 2 cups of water at least 1 hour before you begin to exercise.
- "Cap off your gas tank" by drinking another cup of water 20 to 30 minutes before your workout begins.
- In order to replenish water and maintain hydration, drink about a half of a cup of water every 10 to 15 minutes while you work out. (That equals a few gulps from your water bottle.)
- At the end of your workout, drink at least 2 cups of water.
- When working out first thing in the morning, if caffeinated coffee or tea are part of your morning routine, remember that caffeine has a diuretic effect, speeding up the metabolism of water in your system and minimizing the absorption into your cells. Be sure to make up for unaccounted-for water by upping your intake to 2 glasses of water for every 1 cup of coffee or tea to compensate for this additional water loss.

Water and Weightloss

Diet plans always seem to suggest that you drink a full glass of water when you feel hungry and a full glass just before a meal. Why? Oftentimes we mistake dehydration for hunger. Somehow our mental wires accidentally get

Food Tip

Drink water and juice when flying in an airplane. Caffeine in coffee and colas will dehydrate your body both inside and out.

crossed and that craving for watermelon (which is filled with water) is really a sign that what you actually need is just plain water. Before you indulge in a feeding frenzy, check to make sure that your brain and your stomach are on the same page. Close the refrigerator, put down the fork, and pour yourself a nice tall glass of cold water. Wait a few minutes, since it takes your brain approximately 15 minutes to catch up with your body, and then gauge your hunger pangs. If you still feel hungry, then you really are hungry. Eat!

Splurging

If you happen to splurge—once—don't fear that you have completely sabotaged your program. YOU HAVEN'T! Just get back on track. I have never known a celebrity not to cheat, not to need a sweet once in a while. So it is normal that you might want to devour a cookie or down a slice of pizza. And that is okay. Just remember, balance and moderation is key. But you need to know that it will be hard to be at the top of your game if you do make the decision to splurge. Just be sure to keep your goals in mind. The questions you should be asking yourself are: Where do I want my body to be? When do I want to get there?

If one of my clients has a film that they are shooting in one month, and their body needs to be at its peak, sorry, but I insist on stamping out little indulgences. On the other hand, if they have one year before shooting begins, we have got worlds of time to prepare. You want a slice of cake? Go ahead. Eat your heart out! As long as it is just one piece. Just try and eat your cake after a workout when your body is pumping instead of at midnight when you are about to lie down for eight hours of sleep.

I know, you have always been told not to eat fat and sugar. But why? Imagine this—you've got a fire burning; you pour gasoline atop the wood, fueling the flames. If you keep pouring on that gasoline, the fire will never feel inclined to use the wood for fuel. But once you take away that gasoline, the fire is forced to fend for itself as it desperately attempts to use the wood for fuel. Now imagine that the gasoline is sugar or fried foods and that the wood is your body's fat. Your body is so accustomed to using sugar as fuel that it never needs to dip into your fat deposits for energy. Once that sugar is taken away your body becomes completely confused as it struggles to find another source of energy. Fat puts up the good fight and holds on to your thighs and stomach for dear life until slowly but surely it begins to lose strength.

Nutritional deficiencies can have serious health consequences. Making the right food choices can significantly reduce your risk of developing cardiovascular disease, cancer, and diabetes, while simultaneously improving your energy level, elevating your mood, and boosting your immune system. Good nutrition involves eating enough (but not too much) of the right foods, having regular meals, and staying hydrated in order to get all the nutrients, such as the vitamins, minerals, and protein your body needs to stay healthy. It's a matter of choice!

Educate Yourself

Carbohydrates: carbs are your fuel source.
Protein: for building muscle and muscle repair.
Fat: unsaturated fat (good) . . . saturated fat (not good).

I will give you a list of healthy choice foods that you should become familiar with so that you can make proper choices wherever and whenever, without being burdened by the confusion-inducing nuisance of measuring or calorie counting. I will also give you a variety of meals to choose from, knowing that your own cravings differ from day to day, so you can choose what your palate desires. I do not want to tell you what to eat, I want you to learn how to make your own healthy choices. It's your body, it's your life . . . it's your choice. You are in control—take it.

This system of eating will help you gain more energy, lose fat, and gain lean muscle. You should eat approximately every 3 hours. This will keep your metabolism higher, keep your energy levels up, and minimize your chances of overeating during one large meal.

Once a week, you will need to spend a little time planning and shopping for the right foods. Not being prepared will lead to last-minute choices, which tend to be fast food and junk, which will, in turn, increase fat and decrease muscle. Spending a little time preparing will not only keep you nutritionally sound, it will also save you money. Preparing chicken breasts at home is a lot more affordable than going out to a restaurant, and it gives you the power of preparing meals, therefore knowing exactly what oils and extras you put on them. Preparing your own food makes you that much more in control of your body.

When you learn a few simple concepts of eating right, you will find it to be simpler, more enjoyable, and cost effective. I admit—some fast foods taste really good. But how do you feel after you eat them? Bloated, lacking energy, greasy? That is because you are. Eating poorly makes you bloated, tired, and it even affects your skin. I promise you, this food and exercise program will change your life!

We will keep this system simple while maximizing your intake of proteins, carbs, fats, vitamins, and minerals. You will learn food combinations that will maximize nutritional value and energy. There is a lot to learn about nutrition, and we'll only scratch the surface together. But keep in my mind, you did not buy this book to take a full-on seminar about nutrition. Yes, there are things that I could teach you, intricacies of food that would either confuse or bore you. So I have decided to leave that out. Instead, I want to give you the information that you really need and will put to use in your daily life. Once you become familiar with this new attitude change you can always purchase a book solely on nutrition to further your studies.

Guidelines for Planning Your
New Nutritional Attitude

A. Eat 5 to 6 Meals a Day.

This includes 3 medium-size meals plus snacks in between. In order to keep your metabolism efficiently burning calories, you should be eating approximately every 3 hours. This is not to say that you should have entire meals, but eat something healthy every 3 hours. Getting into this healthy habit will:

- Keep you more alert and increase your concentration.
- Control your appetite. You won't overeat as easily as you might when you eat 3 large meals, knowing you have to wait hours before you eat again.
- Regulate your blood sugar level, maintain an elevated energy level, and minimize mood swings.
- Help build lean muscle mass.
- Raise your metabolism, allowing you to burn more calories.
- Help lose fat. If you eat too few calories, your body thinks you are starving it. In order to conserve calories for energy, it first burns through muscle. We don't want to lose muscle because, if you remember, the more muscle we have, the more calories are naturally burned off. As it is, as we age, the body loses one pound of lean muscle mass every year.

B. Plan Your Meals.

When shopping, make healthy food choices. Shop on the outer aisles of the store, where the fruits, veggies, and meats are. Most of the stuff down the aisles are junk. If you need something down an aisle, leave your cart and walk to it, pick up only what you need, then walk back to the cart. This helps you avoid all temptations. Once you get home, prepare foods for on-the-go moments. Have salads and proteins ready in plastic containers. With options precooked and ready to go, hunger pangs are less likely to make you turn to fast-food junk. There is no excuse to eat junk. A little prep time goes a long way.

Stay hydrated. Connective tissue and joints dry up with age,

Food Tip

Bring food to work/school in Tupperware to minimize your desire to eat unhealthy fast food for lunch. Make healthy eating a priority and take responsibility.

therefore, aging you faster. Keep a case of bottled water around so you always have water on the go. Soft drinks, beer, fruit juices, and sport drinks are heavy in calories and sugar. Water is always the best. When properly hydrated, your urine should be clear, pale, or lemonade-colored. If it is darker, it is usually an indication of dehydration.

C. Be Sure Your Meals Are Balanced.

All meals should contain protein, carbohydrates, good fats, and fiber.

D. Snack Healthfully in between Meals.

When you are not in the mood for a meal, but you need something to snack on, have healthy snacks such as fruits and nuts.

Don't allow your body to dip into a state of hunger. If your stomach is growling, that is a sure sign that your metabolism has slowed and your blood sugar has dropped. The goal is to maintain balance. Eating healthy snacks between meals will help maintain that balance. Green apples with peanut butter, nuts, and protein shakes are great fast foods. When I make protein shakes at home, I blend together water, fruit, protein powder, powdered vitamin and mineral supplements, and flaxseed oil. Delicious and nutritious!

Food Tip

Fresh lemons are an old cure for seasickness. They often prevent morning sickness too. Feeling bloated? Drinking lemon water in the morning can help to de-puff! Sniff fresh lemons, suck wedges plain, or drink lemon-infused water. Experiment to find what is most effective for you.

E. Don't Skip Breakfast.

I am sure you have heard this before and you will hear it again from me—breakfast is the most important meal of the day. Don't skip it! Your body has been deprived of food all night long; in order to jump start it, you need to feed it. If your body does not receive the nutrients it craves, it will automatically go into starvation mode, tightly holding on to its calories and refusing to let your metabolism burn them. In need of a source of fuel, your metabolism will turn to your muscles for energy. You cannot replace breakfast with coffee. Caffeine alone is an artificial and temporary metabolism boost. But it will not prevent the muscle consumption. Eating a balanced meal of protein, carbohydrates, fat, and fiber will raise your metabolism, give you increased energy, and provide fuel for the brain.

A Few Random Food Tips and Suggestions

Meats should be baked, grilled, or broiled, and they should always be lean.

Pasta should be a side dish and not an entire meal.

Brown or wild rice is better than white.

If you must have your soft-drink fix, go with diet or light for fewer calories.

Dilute fruit juice with water to minimize calories. Unsweetened fruit juice is better than the 10 percent juice (that means that the other 90 percent is sugar!).

Reduce your coffee intake to mornings only. If you like cream with your coffee, make it fat-free or low-fat milk. Instead of sugar use Splenda.

Natural, fresh foods are better than frozen and processed.

The list you are about to read is based on the nutritional value of various foods. Of course there are foods not on this chart, and you may eat what you like, but this will give you a good idea of how to make healthy choices.

> ## Food Tip
>
> Eat your meals off an 8-inch plate instead of a 12-inch plate, as this will aid in proper portion control and calorie intake.

Fats

Good

OILS: olive oil (for cooking too), flaxseed oil, canola oil

FRUITS AND VEGGIES: avocado, olives

SEEDS: pumpkin, sunflower

NUTS: almonds, cashews, pecans, walnuts, soy nuts, macadamia (raw)

Fair

LEGUMES: natural peanut butter, peanuts

Poor

DAIRY: butter, cream, cream cheese, sour cream, ice cream, margarine, whole milk

OILS: vegetable shortening, lard

Proteins

Good

FISH/SEAFOOD: anchovies, calamari, cod, flounder, grouper, halibut, mackerel, mahi mahi, salmon, sardines, swordfish, tuna (water-packed), sushi, clams, mussles, crab, lobster, oysters, shrimp/prawns, scallops, swordfish, snapper

POULTRY: chicken (white meat, skinless), ground turkey (extra lean), turkey breast (skinless)

> **Food Tip**
>
> Eat protein within 1 hour after your workout in order to rebuild and repair muscle tissue. This will not bulk your muscles; it will nourish them.

MEAT: buffalo, filet mignon, flank steak, ground beef (93 percent lean), ham (96 percent fat-free), London broil, pork loin (lean), top and bottom round, venison

LEGUMES: black beans, soybeans (edamame)

DAIRY: cheeses (less than 2 percent fat), egg beaters, egg whites, milk (fat-free, skim), yogurt (low-fat/low-sugar)

Fair

POULTRY: chicken (with skin), ground turkey (85–90 percent lean)

MEAT: ground beef (85–90 percent lean), roast beef, duck, turkey bacon, pork chop

LEGUMES: (eaten alone) chickpeas, kidney beans, lentils, pinto beans

DAIRY: cottage cheese (1–2 percent fat), frozen yogurt (low-fat/low-sugar), milk (1–2 percent fat), whole eggs, yogurt (whole milk)

Poor

MEAT: beef (fatty cuts), ground beef (more than 10 percent fat), NY strip, T-bone, bacon, hot dog, pepperoni, salami, liver, pork sausage

DAIRY: hard cheeses, whole milk

Carbohydrates

Good

BREADS: pumpernickel, rye, sourdough

CEREALS: cheerios, Kashi, oatmeal (slow cook, not instant)

STARCHES: brown rice, couscous

VEGGIES: beets, sweet potatoes, yams, broccoli, asparagus, brussel sprouts, cucumbers, field greens, green beans, romaine lettuce, snap peas, spinach, bell peppers, carrots, celery, eggplant, mushrooms, soybeans, squash, tomatoes

FRUIT: apples (green), blackberries, blueberries, cantaloupe, cherries, grapefruit, grapes (red), honeydew, kiwifruit, mangoes, oranges, papaya, peaches, plums, pomegranates, raspberries, strawberries, watermelon

Fair

BREADS AND BAKERY: whole-wheat bread, muffins (wheat or oat)
CEREALS: corn- and rice-based cereals
STARCHES: egg noodles, pasta (whole-wheat or vegetable)
VEGETABLES: potatoes (baked), iceberg lettuce, yellow squash, zucchini
FRUIT: dates

Poor

BAKED GOODS: bagels, cakes, doughnuts, English muffins, white bread
CEREALS: sugar cereals
DAIRY: ice cream, frozen yogurt (sugar)
SALADS: coleslaw, potato salad, creamy salads

Beverages

Good

Tea (decaf-green, black, or white), water, red wine (in moderation)

Fair

Coffee, diet soft drinks, unsweetened fruit juices, caffeinated teas, white wine, orange juice

Poor

Beer, fruit juice, hard liquor, Kool-Aid, smoothies, soft drinks, wine coolers

Condiments

Good

Balsamic vinegar, cayenne pepper, garlic, herbs/spices, horseradish, hummus, mustard, pesto, salad dressing (fat-free), salsa

> **Food Tip**
>
> Remember, in the morning you must eat break
> fast. I actually split the words for a reason, to re-
> inforce that your first meal of the day is breaking
> the fast that your body has just endured as you
> slept. In order to get your metabolism moving
> again, it is essential to break your fast first thing
> in the morning.

Fair

Ketchup, BBQ sauce, salad dressing (low-fat), syrup (light)

Poor

Mayonnaise, Miracle whip, salad dressing, sugar

Preparing meals should not be labor-intensive, requiring a lot of time or money. You can make healthy, tasty choices in minutes.

Below are a few of my favorite meals:

Breakfast Choice Combinations

1. Oatmeal (slow cook). Toppings—cinnamon, fruit (bananas, strawberries, or blueberries). Use 2 percent milk if needed.
2. Egg-white omelet. Optional add-ons: low-fat cheddar cheese, tomato, mushrooms, peppers, onions, chicken, turkey bacon, salsa, seasonings (basil, thyme, black pepper, garlic). Use olive oil or an olive oil spray for cooking.
3. Cereals such as Kashi, Cheerios, All-Bran, Grape Nuts, Special K. Use 2 percent milk. Fruit and a hard-boiled egg.
4. Granola topped with low-fat yogurt and fruit.

You can mix and match these breakfast choices to avoid boredom. If you love eggs for breakfast, experiment with different ways of preparing them: hard-boiled, poached, scrambled, or over easy (but be sure you cook with olive oil or olive oil spray).

If you like to have bread with breakfast, choose multigrain and have only 1 slice. Stay away from eating bread on a daily basis. Coffee in the morning is okay to jump-start your metabolism. I'll admit—I drink it too.

Lunch Choice Combinations

1. Tuna (water-packed) mixed with ½ spoon of mayonnaise and ½ spoon Grey Poupon mustard. Put it on a bed of sprouts or lettuce and avocado. Add your favorite extras, such as pickles, tomato, onion, or an apple on the side.

> **Food Tip**
>
> Use the Bs to cook meat: broil, barbecue, bake, or braise meats, and you will save lots of calories over frying, stewing, and sautéing.

2. Sliced turkey breast atop a mixed green salad and 1 cup of vegetable soup.
3. Chicken strips (not fried), with broccoli and black beans.
4. 2 slices of multigrain bread, lean roast beef, mustard, lettuce and tomato, with a side of green beans and a cup of lentil soup.
5. Grilled chicken breast, and a side of fresh vegetables and yams.

Dinner Choice Combinations

1. Chicken stir fried with steamed vegetables and steamed brown rice.
2. Broiled salmon with a side of steamed brown rice and steamed spinach.
3. Grilled chicken breast, a medium-size baked potato and steamed vegetables.
4. Lean beef with a side of whole-grain pasta and green veggies.

My beverage of choice for every meal is water. It is suggested to drink an entire glass of water before taking a bite of food in order to help fill up your stomach and avoid over eating. Learn to drink water with every meal. Water . . . water . . . water!

Depending on your schedule, here are some options for your daily nutrition:

Food Tip

A small protein shake in the morning is great! It awakens the system and acts as fuel for energy.

Food Tip

Shop the salad bar when you need ingredients for a recipe but don't want to purchase too much. Cheaper!

Food Tip

That eating late is a sure way to pack on the pounds is a myth. It is the type of high-calorie food one chooses while sitting in front of the TV after dinner—ice cream, chips, chocolate—that are likely to make you fat. Be concerned with the kinds of foods you eat, not the clock.

If You Work Out Before Work

6:00 A.M. Nutrition shake or fruit

6:15 A.M. Workout

7:15 A.M. Breakfast: egg-white omelet with veggies, and a small bowl of oatmeal with fruit, and water (plus coffee if you would like)

10:15 A.M. Nutrition shake

1:15 P.M. Lunch: tuna with ½ teaspoon Dijon mustard, ½ teaspoon fat-free mayonnaise, a dash of cracked pepper, sprouts, avocado, and tomato on rye bread or bed of lettuce. Water.

4:15 P.M. Nutrition shake or snack: a green apple with natural peanut butter

7:15 P.M. Dinner: broiled salmon, steamed brown rice, green vegetable. Water.

10:15 P.M. Nutrition shake or snack

If You Work Out During Lunchtime

7:30 A.M.	Breakfast: oatmeal w/fruit, hard-boiled egg
10:30 A.M.	Nutrition shake
1:30 P.M.	Workout
2:30 P.M.	Lunch: grilled chicken, baked potato, fresh vegetables
4:00 P.M.	Nutrition shake or snack
7:00 P.M.	Dinner: lean-cut red meat, spinach, yams
10:00 P.M.	Nutrition shake or snack

If You Work Out After Work

7:00 A.M.	Breakfast: bowl of cereal with fruit
10:00 A.M.	Nutrition shake or snack
1:00 P.M.	Lunch: sliced chicken breast on a bed of lettuce, spinach, tomatoes, handful of nuts, olive oil dressing
4:00 P.M.	Nutrition shake or snack
6:00 P.M.	Workout
7:00 P.M.	Dinner: lean pork chops, vegetables, whole-wheat pasta
10:00 P.M.	Nutrition shake or snack

7

Week One—Let's Do This!

*You cannot discover new oceans unless you
have the courage to lose sight of the shore.*

—UNKNOWN AUTHOR

Wake-up

Try to allow yourself an extra hour in the morning to get your workout in before you start your day. This way you can get it over with and not have to worry about scheduling it in later. I know, the thought of getting up earlier than usual, putting on your exercise clothes and dragging your still-sound-asleep body into the living room to start working it out is probably the last thing that you want to do, especially if you are not an early bird. But believe me, after a few days of forcing your eyelids open, you will soon be craving the adrenaline rush and endorphin release that a solid A.M. workout can give.

For some of you, your eyes refuse to open until a pot of coffee has jump-started your system. If you are one of those people, good! A cup or two first thing in the morning will raise your metabolism and give you that needed kick-start. Just try and chase the coffee with a cup of water to hydrate. If you don't depend on coffee to open your eyes, great! After a few bites of breakfast, you can start working out immediately! Keep your pre-workout meal small and give yourself about an hour before you start to move your body. This allows your digestive system do its work—the digesting. I do suggest that you eat something first thing in the morning to break your fast, hence "breakfast." If cereal or eggs are too much of an ordeal for you, try a mini protein shake first thing in the morning, just to give your body a little fuel to start burning and jump-start your system. Of course, working out at any time of the day is recommended, but morning workouts are best. After a long night sleep, your metabolism is naturally slower when you first wake up, so this will give you that "get up and go" that you need to seize the day. Take full advantage of every waking minute and its calorie-burning potential. Get up and go!!! Accomplishing something first thing in the morning sets the tone, sending you on your way to a productive day. Mentally energized, you will have the capacity to accomplish more and waste less time. You won't sit in the office for 2 hours, guzzling a cup of coffee, waiting for your mind to finally shift into gear. You will already be focused and in full gear!

More than burning more calories and taking full advantage of the lasting energy that early morning workouts can provide, an easy excuse to not exercise is "but I'm too busy today" or "I ran out of time." But getting it over with in the morning minimizes those excuses. Your only excuse in the morning is likely, "but I am too tired," whereas, at night, a multitude of things can come up, pushing back your workout further and further until it is truly too late. You can control your mornings by simply waking up a little earlier. To address the "but I'm too tired" complaint, regular exercise gives you more energy throughout the day and actually makes you need less sleep. It helps you to wake up revitalized, instead of tired and groggy no matter how many hours you slept. If it is important enough, you can surely find a way around the excuses. Find time.

Motivation Through Mantras

I know, affirmations may seem cheesy or arrogant, but the fact is that they work. Sometimes, you have to convince yourself that you are ready for something new in order to move forward to the

Affirmation

"I am in control of my life. I am confident. I am strong and powerful and I deserve to be happy. I am healthy and happy and I feel whole. I am open to change and accepting of greatness."

next level. Repeating a mantra aloud (you can do it alone and use a hushed tone if that makes you more comfortable) each morning has been shown to help rewire a person's mentality, helping to focus on the future and generating a positive outlook on life. A mantra is similar to an affirmation. A mantra is a single word, sound, or phrase of your choice that resonates with you. In other words, it has meaning to you, it motivates you, or it relaxes you. Once you have selected that word, sound, or phrase, you would repeat it in an effort to unite your body and mind. Mantras are often repeated during meditation, when the mind is focused and the breath is slow and controlled. But they can be repeated anytime. I often suggest that you repeat your mantra immediately upon waking up, as you are doing your warm-up before beginning to exercise. Similar to being in a meditative state, as you warm up your muscles, your mind is incredibly connected to your body, and you are acutely aware of your muscles and ligaments and their evolving state of warmth.

Mantras are so powerful that they have been shown to ease stress and lower the respiratory rate. According to the *Journal of Communication,* adopting a positive mantra can help motivate you to take better care of yourself. Repeating a phrase, such as "I am only as old as I feel" may change and improve your view on aging, encouraging the incorporation of healthy habits into your daily life. To make your mantra even more effective, write it down, or type it up, and put it in a place where you will see it often, such as in your wallet, at the foot of your bed, next to your computer, or on your refrigerator. Once you change your perspective on aging and begin to adopt healthy habits, you will, in turn, naturally age slower and feel healthier and younger.

Getting Started

Start on a Monday. Mondays represent a new week, a clean slate, and a fresh start. After a revitalizing weekend, you are more apt and ready to begin anew. Your body will be rested, your mind energized, and you will have an entire week to get off to a great start! In preparation to begin, spend a little time on Sunday organizing your meals and setting out your workout clothing for the next morning, and, finally, remember to set your alarm a bit early in order to make time to exercise—without feeling rushed. Each week will progressively get more intense as we add extra minutes and increasingly difficult exercises to your regimen. After 8 weeks, if you truly stick with me and let me guide you to become your best, you will be well on your way to your perfect body! But it takes serious dedication and determination. A perfect body is not made overnight, nor after one week or even one month. A perfect body comes with consistent hard work and unwavering commitment. While consistency is essential, it is also important not to overdo it. Follow my guidelines. Keep to the schedule and keep your butt moving!

Sundays will be your day off. Why? Because everyone deserves a break once in a while—plus, your muscles need to heal in order to become stronger. It is a strange, yet entirely true concept that as you lift weights your muscles are actually weakening. I know, you probably thought it was the exact opposite, but the fact is that while you exercise, your muscle tissue is tearing and breaking down. *It is while you rest that your muscles repair themselves and become stronger.* That is why it is important to exercise to exhaustion. You want to be weak and fatigued by the end because then your muscles have more recovery, and therefore more strength potential. Of course, if you exercise all of the time, there is no time for your muscles to recover, therefore there is no time for your body to become strong, and you are actually doing yourself a disservice and risking injury. When you work out, work hard. You know the age old adage—"no pain, no gain." Take it to heart. Pain equals change. Embrace the discomfort knowing that you will be stronger because of it. Every drop of sweat and each second that you push your limit brings you closer to your perfect body.

If you think about it, it is through pain that we become stronger people, not just in exercise, but in life. You went through that grueling, sleepless semester in school that, in the end, earned you an A and helped you take the next step to your successes. When your ex-boyfriend (or-girlfriend) stole your heart, broke it in half, and left you feeling absolutely empty inside, you learned how to find strength without him. Many of life's greatest pains build us up to be even better, stronger, more equipped people. Enjoy the journey to your perfect body!

Warm-up

The warm-up eases your body into movement, gently getting your blood flowing. If you leave it out, you are only hindering your ability to succeed. You are, in fact, tempting injury. Physiologically, when you begin to move your body, you call to action your respiratory system, muscle fibers, and metabolism. Your blood begins to surge through your veins, circulating within your brain, joints, and muscles at a faster speed. Since your body needs more oxygen, your breathing quickens. To meet the demands of a faster blood flow, your heart rate increases. The quickly moving blood is routed to your muscles, causing them to slightly swell. With all of your systems increasing in speed, your temperature rises, allowing your muscles to burn through stored sugar and fat, using it as energy, therefore burning more calories. The warmer your body gets, the more lubricated and loose it gets, minimizing your chances of injury and readying it to really work out.

Let me break it down for you. You should gradually warm up your body before working out because:

- Easing your body into movement, your muscles are gradually warmed, therefore increasing your blood temperature, which, in turn, allows for a more efficient and effective calorie burn.
- Enhances your metabolism, assisting in an increased rate of delivery of oxygen to your working muscles.
- Loosens your limbs, which minimizes your risk of injury.
- Increases the speed in which messages are delivered from the brain to the working muscle, allowing for more precise muscle control.

- Lengthens the possible duration of your workout due to the fact that your body had more time to adjust to exercise (instead of shocking it into a sudden run), minimizing the amount of lactic acid lingering in your blood.
- Enhances joint mobility, encouraging an increase in flexibility.
- Mentally prepares you to work out at a greater intensity, as your mind acutely focuses on your body.

Stretch

Stretching is one of the core components of Cardio Barre. It is an essential element that many exercisers often rush through, if they do it at all. Though it is essential, it is not something that you do first. How many of you stretch your legs to "warm up" before actually moving your body and getting your blood pumping? Considering the amount of people I see doing this on a daily basis, I would imagine that most of you do. It is time to break that habit, despite the fact that you have been doing it for years, or you see it done on TV or by other exercisers at the gym. *I absolutely do not recommend stretching before you work out.* It is much safer and more effective to stretch during the workout and again at the end.

When we work out together, you will notice that you are stretching throughout the workout. By contracting the muscle (flexing it) then expanding it (stretching), contracting then expanding, you are strengthening and stretching, therefore avoiding that bulky, stubby muscle look, which we do not want.

After your workout is complete and your muscles are warm, you will again stretch, but this will be a more focused stretch. This final stretch is when you really start to limber up your limbs. Your muscles and tendons are more malleable, allowing for a deep stretch that has longer lasting effects. While obtaining a good stretch is important, it is also important not to force it. If there is even a little bit of tension on your muscles and tendons, you are benefiting from the stretch. Move slowly in and out of the positions. Do not bounce the muscle. Hold each position for 20 to 30 seconds. Don't forget to breathe. As you focus on the stretch, bringing your mind to each muscle, your heart rate slows, your breathing becomes less labored, and your body is brought back to a balanced state. To help slow your mind and begin to cool down your body, it helps to turn on slow, calming music. Spend time stretching; don't just rush through it. The minimum amount of time that you should stretch is 5 minutes. The maximum amount of time is endless.

The Program — Mind Your Body: A New You Resolution

Whether you think you can or whether you think you can't, you're right!
—Henry Ford

You don't need a new year to come around in order to make a "new you resolution." All you need is determination and dedication to make change. Exercise is undeniably a physical experience; but it is also an emotional one. As you burn off excess physical pounds, the emotional pounds are also slowly being shed. Sometimes it is the emotional pounds that hold the physical pounds intact. Stop holding on so tightly, and you will feel less mentally *and* physically encumbered. Don't you want to be happy? I know you do. Let me show you how. Once lighter, emotionally, your happiness will radiate from within, exuding your inner light. Your life will begin to change. People will take notice. As the saying goes "smiles are infectious." Soon, the dream you dream will become the future you desire.

Go confidently in the direction of your dreams. Live the life you have imagined.
—Henry David Thoreau

I know, the journey can, at times, be challenging. The fact is that hard work and discipline can be painful, sometimes even boring. But taking the time to focus on your fitness and health is essential. To alleviate some of the treachery, I will show you how exercise can be enjoyable. The reality is that getting fit is a never-ending journey and there are different plans for different people.

Allow me to guide you along this simple approach to exercise and food that you can stick with for a lifetime. I will teach you how to make healthy food choices that still satisfy your sweet tooth and fill your cravings, without hurting your body and throwing you off track. I will guide you along an eating plan that doesn't involve the word "diet" in the sense of limitations. Instead you will make simple, doable healthy choices without the need for excessive measuring or complicated calorie counting that confuse you to the point of giving up. This is not a fad, but a long-term plan that shapes your body lean and keeps it that way for the long run.

A healthy eating plan, coupled with regular exercise, is the key to weight loss and maintenance, and it can be a cure-all for an unhappy, unfulfilled life. Once you put energy into bettering yourself, better things will naturally come to you. This is where my exercise program gets really good. Of course, many of you want to have an exercise program so that you can lose weight and look attractive. But more than that, an exercise program imbues an undeniable confidence that increases your self-esteem and gives you the courage to better your life beyond just your body. This is where the physical element is conjoined with the mental. Body and mind become one; working together as an unstoppable team. Once that connection takes place, you can achieve anything you want in life. Why do you think mobs of people take yoga? The mind/body connection!

Cardio Barre goes several steps further than this, adding an intense workout that strengthens your body and even further connects your body with your mind. When you work out to the point that you are overcoming your own self-perceived boundaries, seemingly approaching your breaking point, and then going beyond it, you will find a personal pride that no one can take away. This pride has nothing to do with arrogance, but about confidence and the knowing that you deserve the best in life. You deserve complete fulfillment. This energy will radiate from the inside out, creating an unexplainable glow that surrounds you.

I want you to get everything you desire out of life, living each day to the fullest with a big smile on your face. I know, the gains seem to be much greater than the amount of energy that you have to put into it. After all I am "just" teaching you about how to eat healthfully and exercise. But that is exactly what is so great about this system. Ask my student Kaden, 53, who, through Cardio Barre, eased arthritis and found the courage to leave an unhealthy relationship, go back to school, and find a fulfilling career; Deborah, who defeated type II diabetes; Loretta, who lost 10 dress sizes and gained confidence; or Scilla, who realized that she truly deserved to be happy and, after years of marriage, left her husband to follow her passions. My students change more than their dress sizes through Cardio Barre—they change their lives. So can you. The exercises in this book can be done anywhere—your living room, bedroom, garage, outside, in an office, in a hotel, at the gym, or even in your kitchen. Open yourself to happiness, and it will come.

MOVE YOUR BODY: WEEK ONE–3 DAYS, 20 MINUTES

The sections in this first week will include:

Warm-up

Pliés

Torso Twist

Upper Body

Stretch

This first week will be very physically challenging. After the first day, your muscles will burn and your body will feel painfully stiff. DON'T LET THAT STOP YOU. You have got to work out on day two in order to get the blood rushing to those sore spots, nourishing those areas and pushing out lactic acid build-up (the source of the sore muscle).

Are you ready to get started?

Day one. We are at the beginning, the beginning of your new, healthier life. Remember, this is not just an exercise program; it is a lifestyle. We are not just dieting and exercising, but we are changing the way you view your life. You have the power to create your own reality as you want it to be. I am your personal coach. It is time to start you on your way to fulfilling your dreams, turning them into reality! A coach is not just a personal trainer, but an adviser—at times a therapist, a motivator, and a friend. I will help you along this path to success. I am here to answer your questions before you ask them, giving you praise and encouragement. But you will ultimately be the one to take yourself to success. You will feel proud and confident of your accomplishments.

You have made it this far in this book. That shows me that you are ready to embrace this change. That you want it so badly you can picture your new life, you can see your new body, you have already mentally gone on a shopping spree for a brand-new wardrobe to fit the soon-to-be-slimmer you! Congratulations! You have already found success. Let's get some more.

Yes, it may be a little scary at times. It may also, at times, be hard. But a little effort and desire in making small changes, one step at a time, will get tremendous results. I wrote this book for you, because I know that you deserve to be happy. Follow me through my 8-week program and I will teach you to eat smarter, redefine your body, and feel fantastic!

Let's start on a Monday. Mondays are perfect days to begin because you are starting the week anew. You had a weekend to relax, rejuvenate, mentally and physically prepare. For this first week, we will work out 3 days, 20 minutes each day. More than exercise, we will slowly adjust your diet so that you are making healthier choices, which will give you more energy and support your new lifestyle.

Before we begin, make sure that you have read the "Terms and Proper Placement" (page 49) section to familiarize yourself with some of the shorthand names of the movements. This will allow you to go immediately to that position with proper placement. The more you review the section, the more familiar you will become.

For the workout, every movement in each section will flow through into the next movement. Imagine a dance. While dancing, you wouldn't constantly stop and start after each movement—that would make for a rather jerky dance. Though this is not a dance

Fit Tip

Take the stairs instead of an escalator or elevator. Burn more calories! Get into a fitness frame of mind . . . always think fit.

class per se, there is an innate fluidity that you should try to follow. You may be a bit jerky at first as you become acquainted with the exercises. But soon you will be able to go with the flow.

There will be a couple of different exercise routines within some sections. You may add a new section as you progress in your strength and ability. Do not try all of the sections right away. Ease your body into it. To change it up, break up a few of the sections to keep your interest and maintain a degree of newness each day. You will activate your mind and increase your awareness of each body part. Cardio Barre begins with your understanding of body mechanics through movement and ends with the integration of your body and mind. Do not rush the moves. Stay in control and you will notice that your workouts will be finished before you know it, leaving you sweat-soaked and strong!

−Warm-up−

Never stretch a cold muscle! Warming up your muscles before a workout will prevent injury to the muscles and joints. The first section focuses on warming up the entire body and slowly bringing up your heart rate. Pick some music that will really get you moving. Turn it up! Feel the music pumping through your blood. We will begin at the barre (or any other hip-height sturdy surface). *Be sure to keep to the order of exercises that I have laid out for the warm-up. They are selected in a certain sequence for a reason.* We will work our way up, warming up every muscle so that when it is time to move into the cardio portion, your body is warm and all of your muscles respond easily and correctly, therefore avoiding injury.

BACK ROLL/RELEASE

■ Face the barre and place both hands on it. Don't grip your hands! Place them. The barre is not there to hold you up—it is there to help you maintain balance.

■ Your legs should be shoulder-width apart.

■ Your arms should be stretched straight (but not locked at the elbows), so that you have about a foot distance between your body and the wall.

■ With straight legs, bend at your waist and lower your body into Flat Back position (see page 49), extending your arms away from the barre.

■ Your butt should be sticking out.

■ Your legs are perpendicular to the floor and your body is parallel, creating a 90-degree angle with your body.

■ Hold your abs in—don't simply suck them in, you need to tighten them.

■ Keep your spine straight and your head in line with your spine, in other words, look down to the floor without completely releasing your head down.

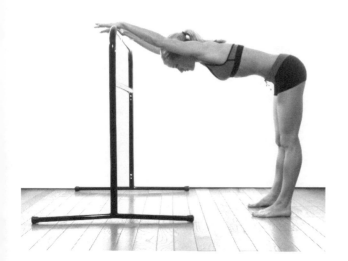
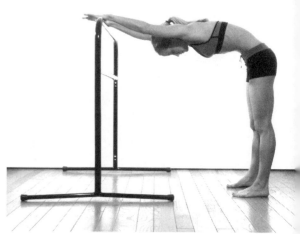

■ You will warm up your back by rolling up through the spine.

■ Start at your lower back and begin to curve each vertebra, rounding through to the top of your spine all the way to your neck and head.

■ Your back should be shaped like a sideways C, with the opening facing the floor, and your neck slightly tucked.

■ Now, reverse the position, arching your back, vertebra by vertebra, creating a U shape with your spine. Slightly arch your neck and head up to the sky.

■ Now release your neck and return to Flat Back.

■ Repeat this 4 times slowly.

■ (Do not pause, move right into the next exercise.)

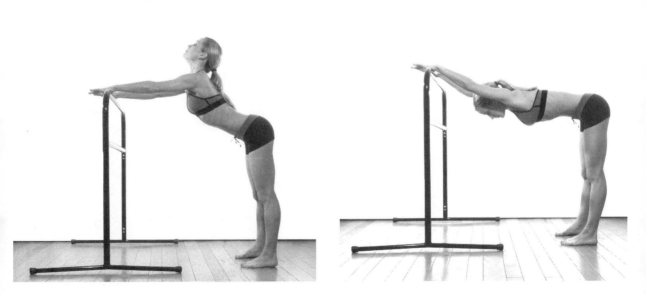

BACK CONTRACTION

- Stay in the Flat Back position and do little back contractions by lifting your lower abs up into your spine, and rounding your lower back as though your abs are pushing your back slightly up to the sky.

- Release to Flat Back.

- Repeat 4 times.

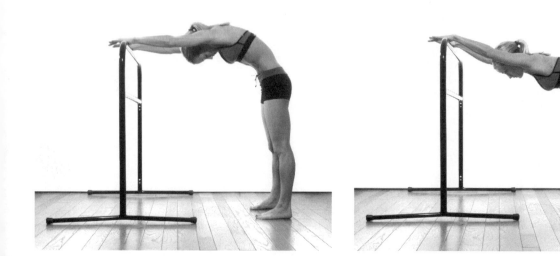

SHOULDER STRETCH

■ Still in a Flat Back position, relax your shoulders and press the weight of your upper torso into your left shoulder and then the right, alternating each shoulder. The movement originates in your waist. Be sure to keep your body below your waist perfectly still.

■ This stretch targets your back and shoulders.

■ Stretch side to side 8 times.

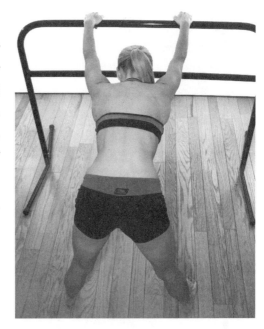

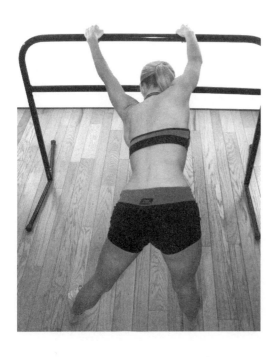

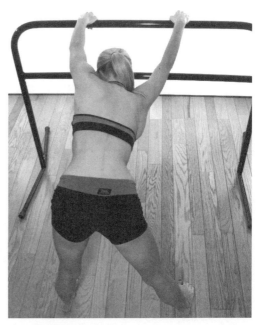

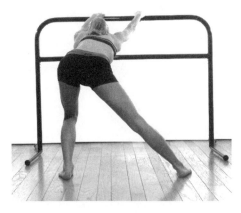

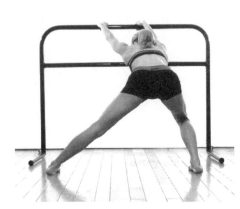

LUNGE STRETCHES

■ To warm up your hamstrings, stand up straight, place your feet two shoulder lengths apart. Be sure that your toes are pointing toward the wall. Bend your right knee, but keep your left knee straight, and lunge over the right leg.

■ Be sure that your knee does not go beyond your toes.

■ Now press through to the other side, bending your left knee and keeping your right knee straight.

■ Alternate back and forth 8 times.

■ To warm up your inner thighs, we will be doing the same position, but turn your feet out (see page 49, Turnout) so that, if they were together, they would be in the shape of a V.

■ Lunge back and forth, alternating legs, 8 times.

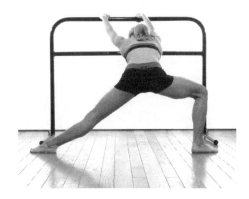

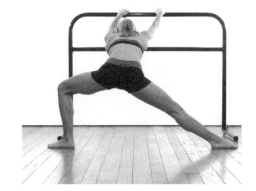

BEND AND STRAIGHTEN

■ Turn your feet back to parallel, toes facing the wall. Bend your back into Flat Back, parallel to the floor. Slowly bend and straighten your knees. In order to protect your knees, be sure that your kneecaps do not pass the front of your toes.

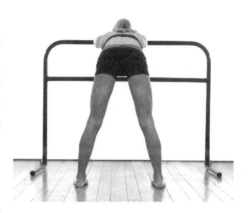

■ Repeat 4 times.

■ Straighten your legs and move your torso over to your right side, pressing your chest onto your right thigh.

■ Release your right arm from the barre and reach it behind you, toward the ceiling.

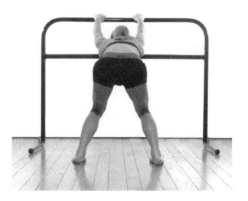

■ Hold for 8 seconds.

■ Return your arm to the barre.

■ Switch sides, pressing your chest onto your left leg.

■ Release your left arm from the barre and reach it behind you, toward the ceiling.

■ Hold for 8 seconds.

■ Return your torso to the center.

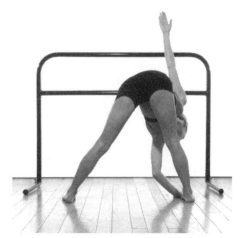

■ Release your arms, head, and neck.

■ Stretch down as far as you can while keeping your legs straight.

■ Roll up to Standing Posture (see page 50).

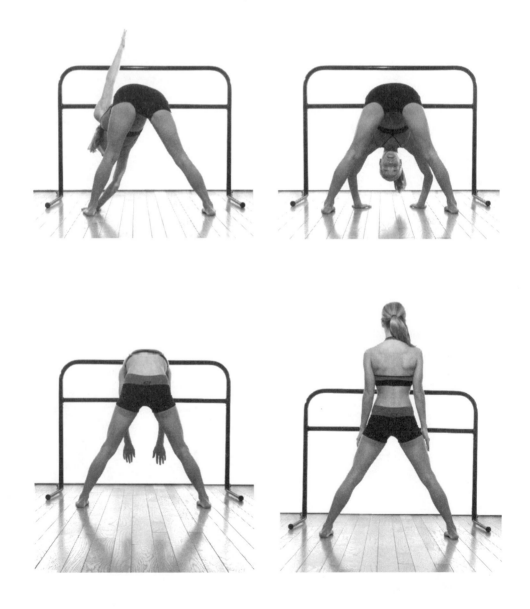

FLAT BACK STRETCH—DOUBLE COUNT

■ Place your right hand on barre.

■ Spread your legs apart so that they are slightly wider than shoulder width.

■ Keep your knees straight and press your torso down to a Flat Back, so that your torso is parallel to the floor.

■ Hold your left arm out to the side, slightly bending at the elbow.

■ Hinge at your waist, allowing your chest to fall forward to the ground, and reach your left arm straight through your legs at knee level.

■ Hold your abs tight and keep your spine straight—from your waist to the top of your head.

■ Pulse your arm through your legs twice. Do not bounce on the muscle, but gently press on the muscle.

■ Stand up straight and return your left arm to the side.

■ Repeat 4 times.

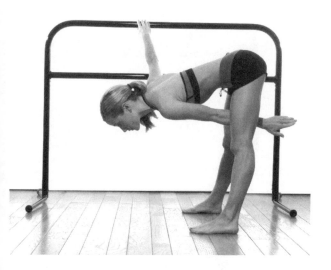
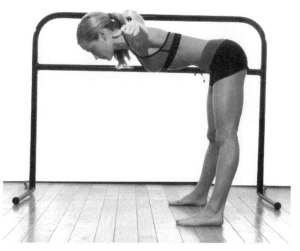

FLAT BACK STRETCH—SINGLE COUNT, BENT KNEES

■ Repeat the Flat Back stretch, but instead of pulsing twice, you will reach your arm through your legs as you bend your knees.

■ As you reach through, stay in a Flat Back position with your abs in.

■ Repeat 8 times.

■ Hold in Flat Back with your left arm reaching out to your side for several seconds.

■ Roll up to standing position.

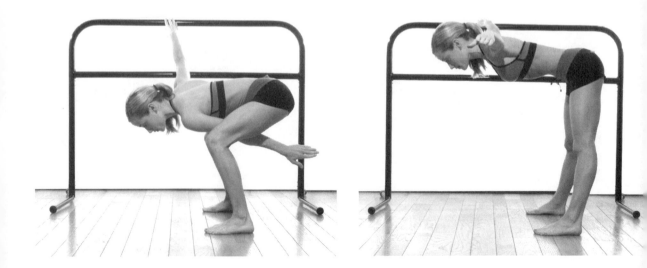

ARM STRETCH

■ Stand up straight.

■ Keep your feet spread slightly more than hips width apart and reach your left arm straight up toward the right corner of the ceiling.

■ Keep your elbow straight, extending your arm as high as possible without lifting your shoulders up to your ears.

■ Alternate arms—reach your right arm straight up to the left corner of the ceiling.

■ Repeat each side 16 times to lengthen the muscles in your arms and torso.

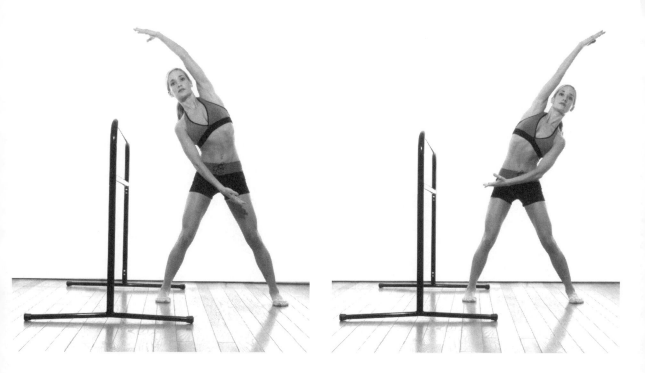

WALK IN PLACE

■ Face your torso toward the barre.

■ Walk in place 16 times at a fast pace to increase your heart rate and get your blood pumping.

■ Hold still.

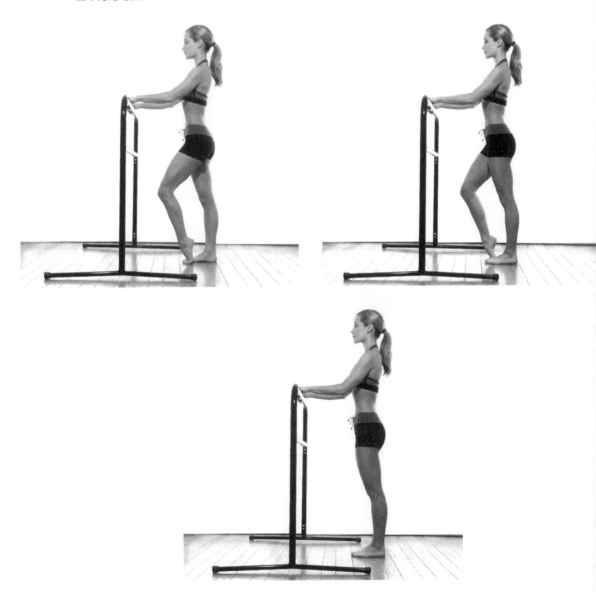

HEEL LIFTS

■ Gently place both hands on the barre.

■ Put your feet together, facing the barre.

■ Stand straight, with your spine elongated and shoulders down.

■ Lift both heels together by pressing over the balls of your feet. (Do not go all the way up onto your toes.)

■ Be sure that you press straight up. Do not press over the outsides of your feet.

■ Lower your heels to the floor without bouncing them down.

■ Concentrate on using your feet and calves to control the lift.

■ Repeat 32 times to strengthen and tone your ankles and calves.

■ Stronger ankles will support your body better when wearing those sexy high-heeled shoes, preventing twisted ankles and injury.

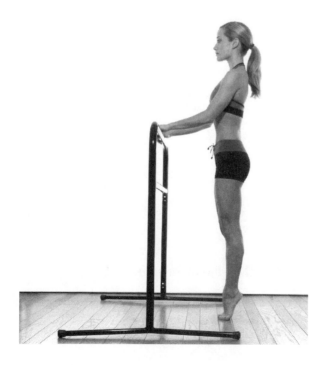

HAMSTRING STRETCH

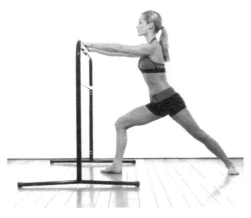

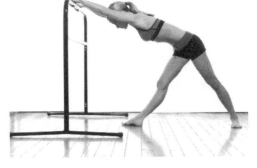

- Face your torso to the barre.

- Gently place both hands on the barre.

- Place your right leg about a foot and a half in front of your left.

- Turn out both feet to a 45-degree angle from the wall.

- Be sure that both heels are on the floor.

- Keep your left leg straight behind you.

- Lunge (bend) your right knee forward so that your knee is over your toes.

- Maintain a center of weight between both legs, so that your torso is upright.

- Hold for 8 seconds.

- Straighten the front leg so both legs are straight.

- Hinge at your hips, press your chest over your right thigh to stretch the hamstring.

- Hold for 8 seconds.

- Straighten up to Standing Position.

- Repeat 4 times.

- Switch legs and repeat on the other side.

−Pliés−

Pliés tone the legs, tighten and lift the butt.
Let's start with a Grand Plié!

GRAND PLIÉ

■ Place your right hand on the barre.

■ Open your legs wider than shoulder width.

■ Turn your feet slightly out to a 45-degree angle.

■ Keep your knees pointing over your toes.

■ Your left arm should be out to your side and slightly bent at the elbow, creating a forward curve.

■ Never work with the arm behind the shoulder. You will compromise the integrity of the shoulder and may cause injury.

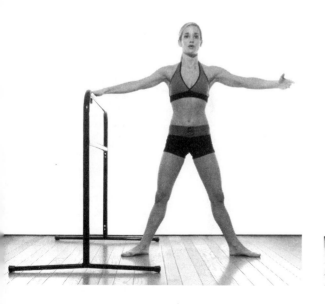
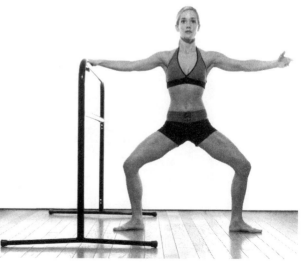

- Plié down by bending your legs while thinking about keeping your torso lifted straight and high.

- Once you have reached the bottom of the Plié (don't allow your butt to dip below your knees), straighten your legs up by squeezing your butt.

- As you push to standing, press from your heels and squeeze your glutes (butt muscles).

- Keep your spine straight and abs in.

- Hold your chest out and shoulders back.

- These are deep, slow Pliés.

- Do 16 slow and controlled repetitions.

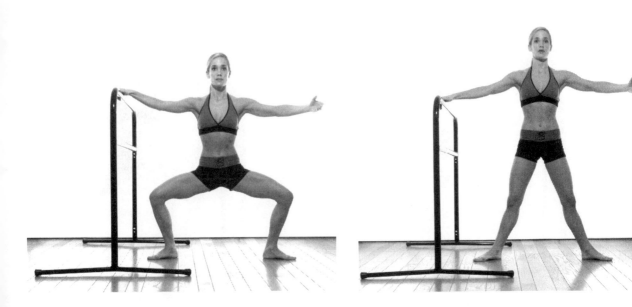

BABY PLIÉ

■ Repeat the same body position and action as the Grand Plié, but this time, press down into the Plié and only come halfway up.

■ You will not be fully straightening your legs.

■ Pick up the tempo and do these at double-time the Grand Pliés.

■ Do 16 reps.

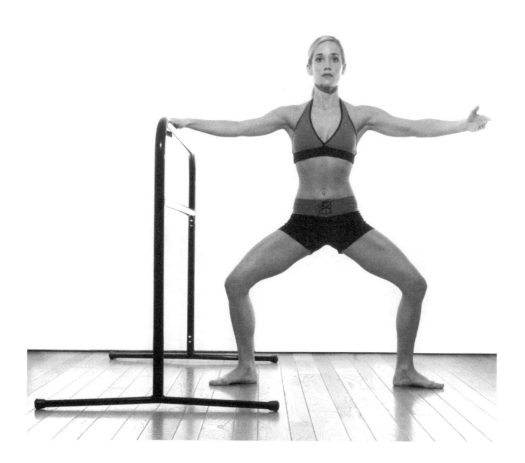

HEEL RISE A

■ Hold the Plié in the bent-leg position and press up through your feet, pushing your heels off the floor, until you are on the balls of your feet.

■ This is not a bouncing action. In fact, your torso and head height should remain at the same level throughout this exercise.

■ Maintain the bend in your knees.

■ Lower your heels back down to the floor so that your feet are flat on the floor.

■ Do 16 reps to strengthen your calves and ankles and improve the arches of your feet.

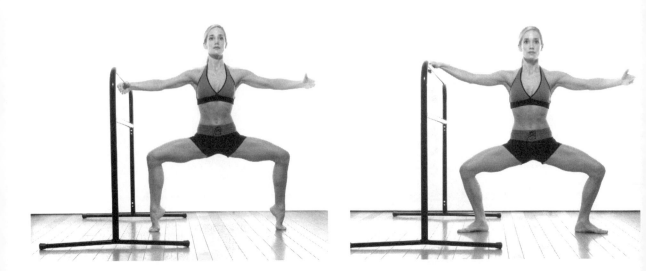

HEEL RISE B

■ Now repeat the entire exercise up on your toes, bending and straightening your knees.

■ The lower you bend your knees, the higher you lift your heels by pressing all the way over the balls of your feet.

■ Do 16 reps.

BALANCE

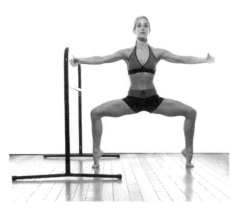

- Hold in Plié (knees bent, balancing on the balls of your feet).

- Take your right hand off the barre.

- Lift both arms, with slightly curved elbows, out to the side.

- Hold for balance.

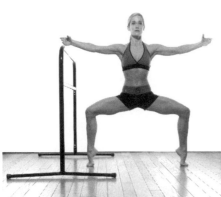

- Lift your arms overhead, creating an oval with your arms. Keep you arms slightly in front of your head. You should be able to see your pinky fingers in your eye line.

- Straighten your legs.

- Hold for balance. In time, your balance will improve as the muscles grow stronger and you learn to find and use your center.

- Lower down.

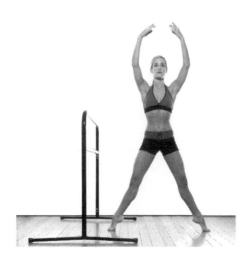

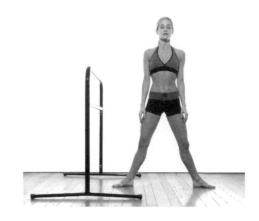

–Other Side–

GRAND PLIÉ

■ Place your left hand on the barre.

■ Place your heels together.

■ Turn out your feet creating a V from heels to toes. Your knees should be directly over your toes.

■ Keep your abs in and spine straight with chest lifted and shoulders pulled back.

■ Plié your knees down, keeping your heels on the floor.

■ Press up to straight leg–heels still on the floor.

■ Do 16 slow, controlled reps.

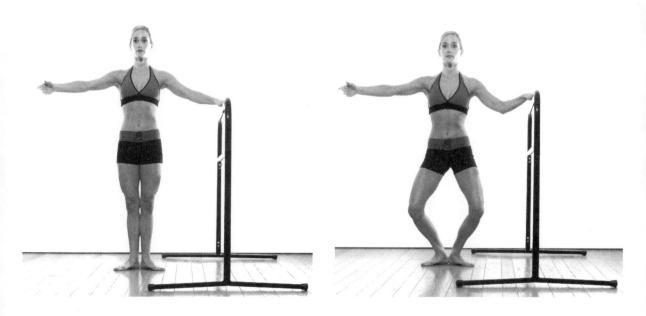

BABY PLIÉ

■ Repeat the same body position and action as the Grand Plié.

■ But this time, press down into the plie and only come halfway up.

■ You will not be fully straightening your legs.

■ Pick up the tempo and do these at double-time the Grand Pliés.

■ Do 16 reps.

HEEL RISES

■ Stay in Plié with bent legs, heels touching, and toes pointing out at a 45-degree angle.

■ Lift your heels only, by pressing over the balls of the feet. Do not raise onto your toes.

■ Lower your heels to the floor, keeping your knees bent.

■ Do 16 reps of heel rises.

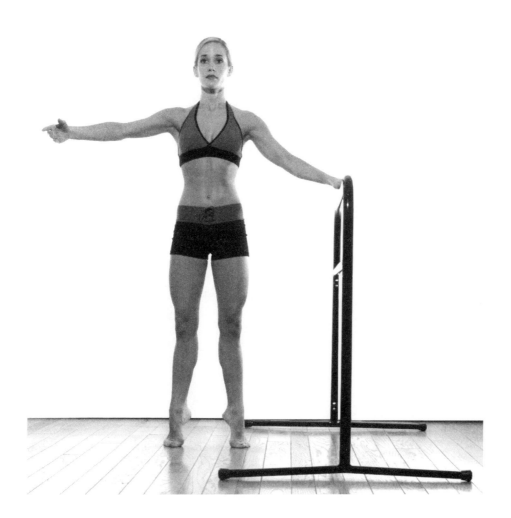

GRAND PLIÉ ON TOE

■ Repeat the Grand Pliés, but this time, stay on your toes.

■ Do 16 reps.

BABY PLIÉ ON TOE

■ Repeat the Baby Pliés, but this time on your toes.

■ Do 16 reps.

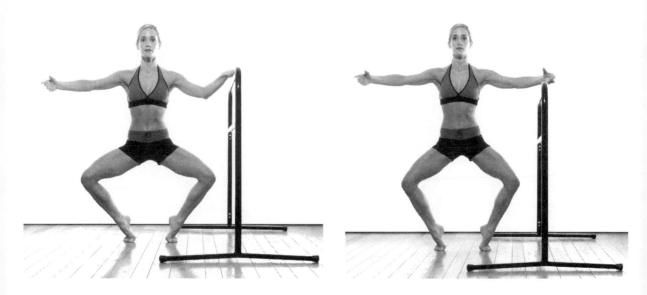

BALANCE

- Hold the Plié in the bent-knee position, balancing on your toes.

- Take your left hand off the barre and hold for balance for a few seconds.

- Straighten your legs and hold your balance on toe.

- Bring your arms over your head in an oval shape for a few seconds.

- Balance.

- Lower down.

- (Increase the amount of reps as desired.)

Fit Tip

The harder you squeeze the legs and buttocks on the way up, the harder your butt will become.

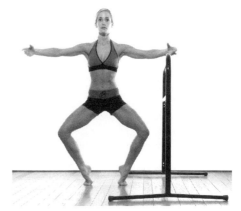

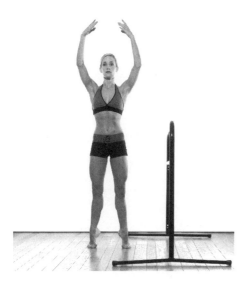

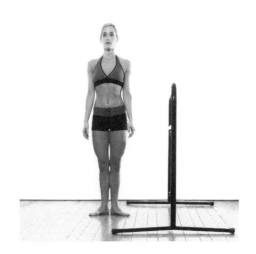

−Torso Twist−

Torso Twists (see page 50) will help trim your waistline. It will take a few attempts before you perfect your technique, but don't give up. Practice makes perfect, and this exercise is very effective in targeting the waist. Many of these exercises also develop coordination and muscle isolation. The movements are continuous and they flow together. Don't stop until the end of the section. The more you do it, the better the fluidity in your movement will become.

BASIC TORSO TWIST

■ Step away from the barre and face a mirror if you have one. (It is always better to work in front of a mirror to observe your placement and watch your muscles at work!)

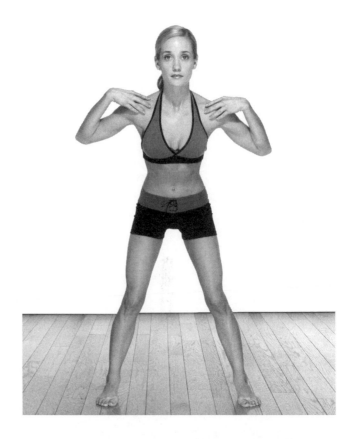

■ Open your legs wider than shoulder width apart.

■ Bend your knees.

■ Lean slightly forward without arching your back.

■ Place your right hand on your right shoulder and left hand on your left shoulder.

■ Allow your elbows to raise a few inches from your chest.

■ Twist your torso to the left so your chest faces the left diagonal.

■ Now twist your torso to the right side of the room.

■ Keep your hips still and twist your upper body only. Your entire torso should change direction, facing front, side, front, side, etc. Keep a steady pace in the movement.

■ Twist for 32 reps.

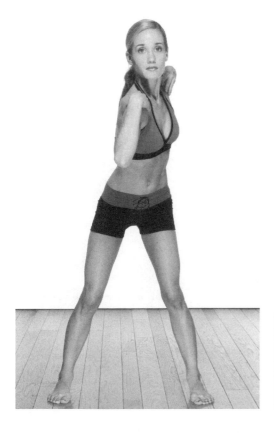
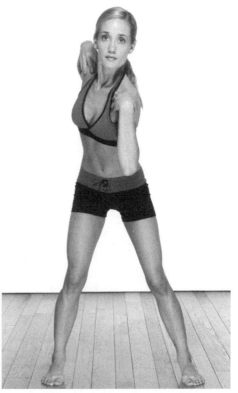

PRESS TWIST

■ Keep your feet in the same position.

■ Place your left hand on your hip.

■ Bend your right arm and hold your right hand up at your right shoulder.

■ Flex your right hand open, facing the mirror in front of you.

■ Press and extend your right hand toward the left side of the room.

■ Extend your arm as far away as you can, slightly rotating your torso to the left.

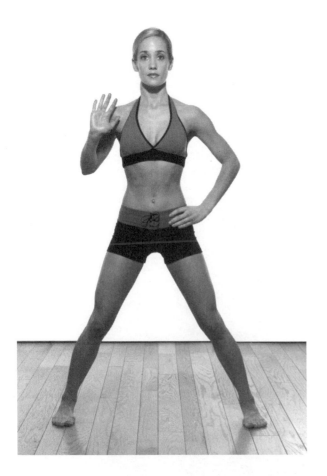
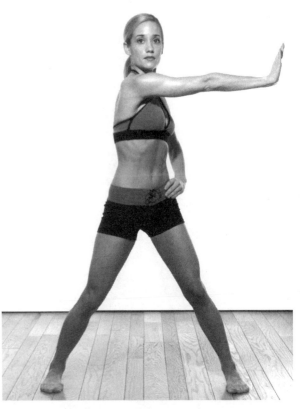

■ Return it to the starting position. (This is not a punch. Imagine that you are pressing through water, or pushing something away from you. This is a resistance move. Squeeze the muscle as you push your arm away from you.)

■ Press forward for 32 reps.

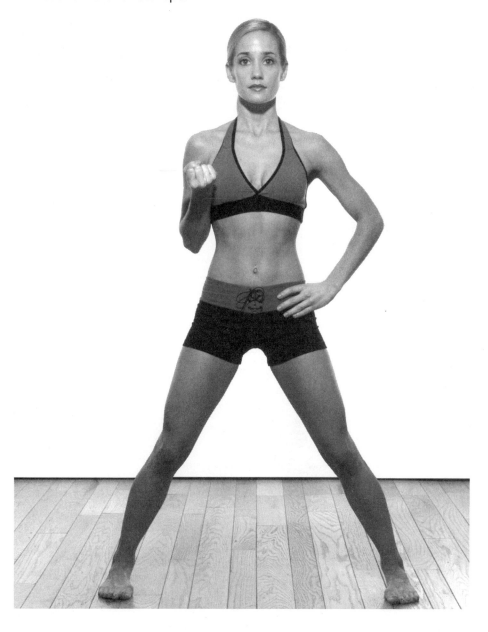

PULL TWIST

■ Maintain the same position, but this time, reach your right arm to the left corner and imagine that you are grabbing something and pulling it toward your right shoulder. (Do not yank your arm. Remember that the focus is always on the torso twisting.)

■ Return your arm to the extended position and repeat the motion.

■ Pull back for 32 reps.

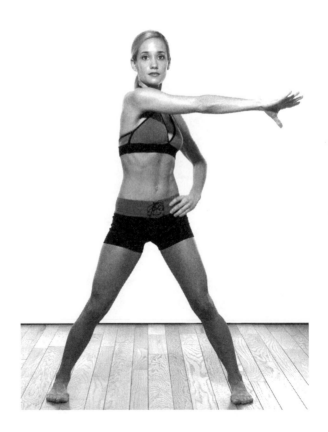

BASIC TORSO TWIST

■ Return to the center and repeat the Basic Torso Twist for 16 reps.

—Other Side—

■ Repeat the exercise using your left arm.

PRESS TWIST

■ Keep your feet in the same position.

■ Place your right hand on your hip.

■ Bend your left arm and hold your left hand up at your left shoulder.

■ Flex your left hand open, facing the mirror in front of you.

■ Press and extend your left hand toward the left side of the room.

■ Extend your arm as far away as you can, slightly rotating your torso to the right.

■ Return it to the starting position.

■ Press forward for 32 reps.

PULL TWIST

■ Maintain the same position, but this time, reach your left arm to the right corner and imagine that you are grabbing something and pulling it toward your left shoulder. (Do not yank your arm. Remember that the focus is always on the torso twisting.)

■ Return your arm to the extended position and repeat the motion.

■ Pull back for 32 reps.

BASIC TORSO TWIST

■ Return to the center and repeat the Basic Torso Twist for 16 reps.

BENT TORSO TWIST

■ Maintaining the same basic stance with your elbows bent at the waist and your hands flexing up at your shoulders, slightly hinge your body forward at your waist so that your back is flat and at a 45-degree angle.

■ Press your right arm past your left knee.

■ Return it to the starting position.

■ Alternate arms—left, right, left, right, etc.

■ Remember to continue to twist from your waist, rotating your torso.

■ Stay hinged over and twist for 32 reps.

FLAT BACK HOLD

■ Hinge into a Flat Back and hold your arms out to your side.

■ Hold.

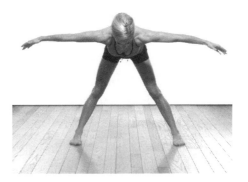

■ Release your body over to the floor, hanging momentarily.

■ Slowly roll up to a standing position.

■ This torso twist section should take approximately 3–5 minutes to complete. You may increase the length of this routine by adding more reps in each subsection. The longer you go, the more cardio you do, the more calories you burn, the more fat you melt away. (NOTE: Make sure you keep the twist in the front of your body working your abs. Do not twist all the way around through the back. Overtwisting could injure your lower back.)

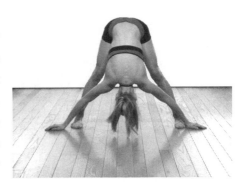

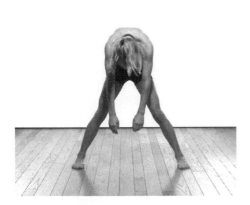

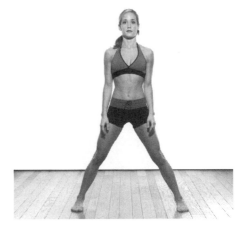

−Upper Body−

−Upper Body Option One−

Engaging your upper body will strengthen and tone your arms, chest, back, and torso while building muscle and burning fat. I am giving you two options for the upper body section. For the first few weeks, I would not advise that you try to do both options in the same workout. Begin with one option, then, as you get better conditioned, add exercises from the other option. Or, if you prefer, you may do one option one day and the other option on another day. There will be many options for you within the framework of this workout so that you can devise your own routine to fit your needs and keep you from getting bored.

TRICEPS ISOLATION

■ Hold a 1-pound weight in your right hand (if you do not have a weight, improvise and use a bottle of water or can of soup).

■ Lunge toward the barre with your left leg forward and your right leg behind you.

■ Place your left hand on the barre.

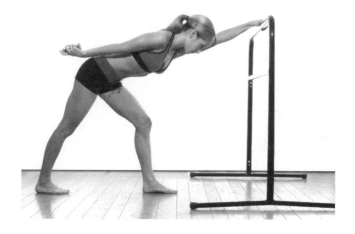

■ Hinge your body into a Flat Back position.

■ Keep your abs in and tight.

■ Lift your right arm so that it is straight alongside your torso, parallel to your back.

■ Maintain a light grip on the weight with your palm facing up.

■ Keep your right arm close to your body.

■ Lift the weight up and down, always raising above waist level—never lower the weight below it. This will isolate and strengthen the back of the arm (triceps).

■ Lift for 32 reps with a straight arm.

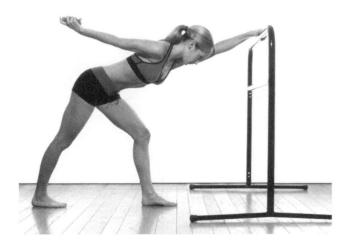

TRICEPS KICKBACK

■ Maintain your body position, but bend your right elbow and bring the weight to your shoulder. When bending your elbow, be sure to keep the upper half of your arm parallel to your back. Only change the positioning of the lower arm as you squeeze the muscle bent and straight. Be careful not to jerk your arm. This is a controlled movement with no impact on the joints.

■ Extend your arm straight again, alongside your torso.

■ Do 32 reps.

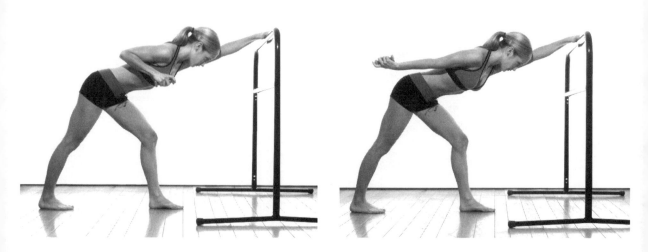

−Other Side−

TRICEPS ISOLATION

■ Switch sides, placing the 1-pound weight in your left hand.

■ Lunge toward the barre with your right leg forward and your left leg behind you.

■ Place your right hand on the barre.

■ Hinge your body into Flat Back position.

■ Keep your abs in and tight.

■ Lift your left arm so that it is straight alongside your torso, parallel to your back.

■ Maintain a light grip on the weight with your palm facing up.

■ Keep your right arm close to your body.

■ Lift the weight up and down, always raising above waist level—never lower the weight below it. This will isolate and strengthen the back of the arm (triceps).

■ Lift for 32 reps with a straight arm.

TRICEPS KICKBACK

■ Maintain your body position, but bend your left elbow and bring the weight to your shoulder.

■ Extend your arm straight again, alongside your torso.

■ Do 32 reps.

■ When lifting weights you want to aim to develop a burning sensation in the muscle. Your goal is to break the muscle down, fatigue it, and allow it to repair itself, growing back stronger. As your strength increases, you may add more reps and increase the weight. For example, try a 2-pound weight instead. You will not bulk up. You will only get leaner, tighter, and sexier.

■ Now let's work some of the other muscle groups!

■ Put the weights down and we will go to the floor.

PUSH-UPS

■ If you have hardwood floors, place a mat or a towel on the floor to add a little cushion.

■ Place your hands shoulder-width apart on the floor.

■ Stretch your body flat against the floor until you find footing and balance on your toes.

■ You will only have your hands and toes touching the floor. The rest of your body will be balancing between. Keep your body straight. Do not stick your butt into the air.

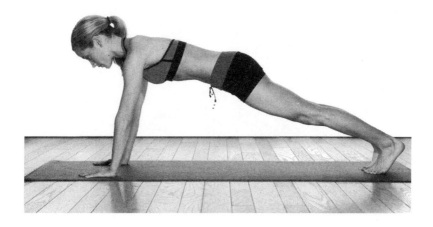

■ Slowly bend your arms, lowering your body a few inches from the floor.

■ Straighten your arms and return to the starting position.

■ Go slow and maintain a constant resistance on your muscles.

■ Repeat until your muscles fatigue.

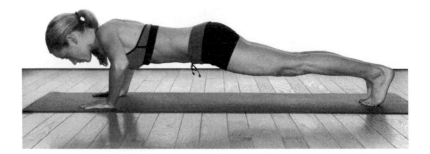

BENT KNEE PUSH-UPS

■ If you find the regular push-ups to be too difficult, start with these.

■ Place your hands shoulder-width apart on the floor.

■ Bend your knees and pull your heels toward your butt.

■ Keep the weight of your body on the front of the knees and not directly on the kneecap.

■ Continue with the push-up motion.

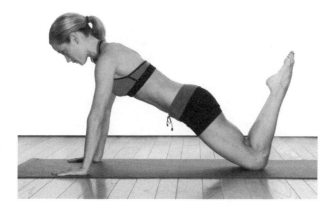
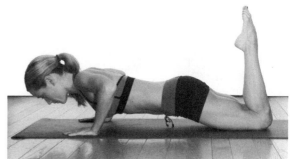

INCLINE PUSH-UPS

■ Stand up against a counter top or couch.

■ Choose an object that is sturdy and can support your weight.

■ Place both hands against it, shoulder-width apart.

■ Your body will be approximately at a 45-degree angle with the floor.

■ These push-ups will seem easier than regular push-ups because you are not supporting your entire body weight. They are great to do anywhere.

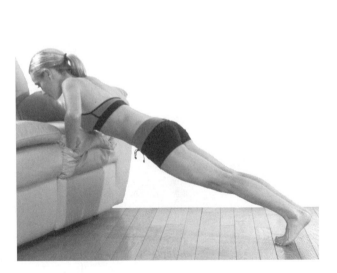

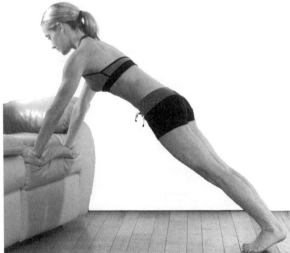

DECLINE PUSH-UPS

■ For a more challenging push-up, place your hands shoulder-width apart on the floor.

■ Rest your feet on a bench or chair approximately 2 feet from the floor. Your weight will be balanced between your toes and your hands. You will feel the stress more in the shoulders and upper chest.

■ In order to constantly keep your muscles guessing, experiment with each of the varying push-up options. You can also try variations within each exercise. If you open your arms wider than your shoulders you will target your chest,

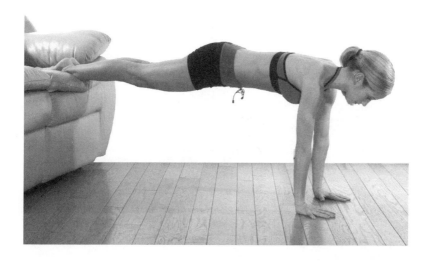

working your pectoral muscles. If you bring your arms in close together you will target your triceps. This way, you will target different muscle groups and allow the others to rest.

◼ On average, do 3 sets of your chosen push-up, with 10 reps in each set. You can vary the amount of reps to fit your fitness level, but always work to challenge yourself. This is not the time to look for the easy way out.

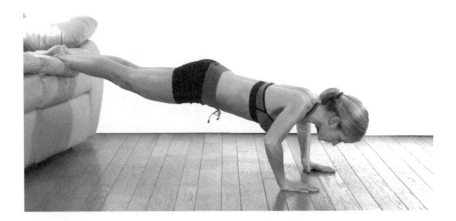

—Upper Body Option Two—

DOWNWARD ARM EXTENSIONS

■ Stand up straight with your feet wider than shoulder-width apart.

■ Slightly bend your knees forward and hinge your body forward 45 degrees.

■ Keep your chest out and head up.

■ Place one weight in each hand, gripping them with palms faced down. (You will work both weights simultaneously.)

■ Hold your arms straight out to your sides. Be sure that they are not behind your shoulders, but instead placed slightly in front of your shoulders. Keep your elbows in line with your shoulders but never higher than them.

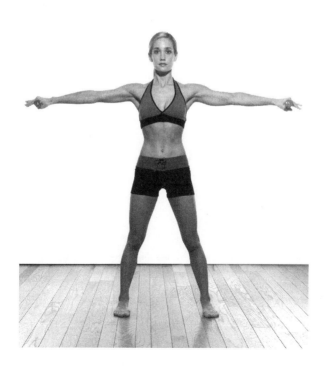

■ Bend your elbows and bring the weights into your rib cage, squeezing instead of dropping.

■ Extend your arms back out, stretched to your sides. (The movement is a press-and-squeezing motion. Do not jerk your arms. The movement should be gentle on the joints.)

■ Do 32 arms extensions to develop your shoulders and back.

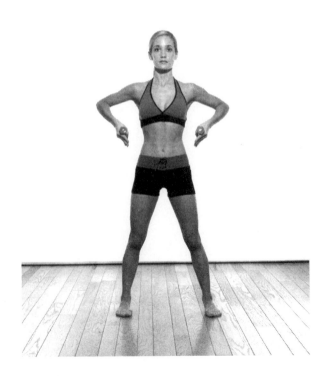

CENTER ARM EXTENSIONS

- Stay in the same position with your torso slightly hinged and your arms straight out to your sides.

- This time, you will turn your palms in so that they are facing your body. It is only a minimal change, but it makes a significant difference as it works different muscles.

- Bring the weights in to your chest with your palms facing your body.

- Press your hands back to the side extension.

- Repeat the center arm extensions 32 times.

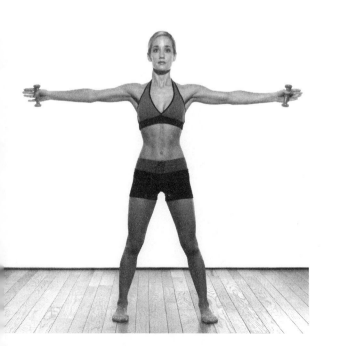
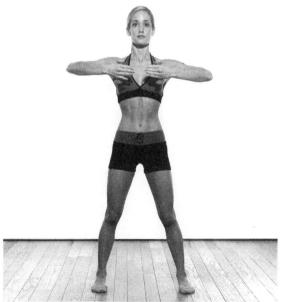

UPWARD ARM EXTENSIONS

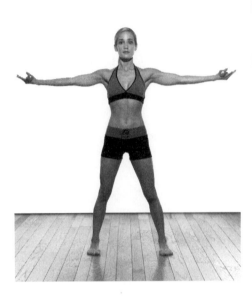

■ Stay in the same Standing Position, with your arms extended out to your sides.

■ Rotate your palms so that they face up to the sky.

■ Bend your elbows and press your forearms up toward your ears. Your elbows should remain even to your shoulder level and parallel to the ground. Only your forearms should be moving.

■ Press your arms back to the straight side extension.

■ Squeeze up and down for 32 reps to isolate the bicep muscles.

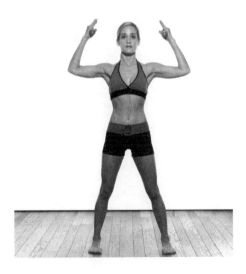

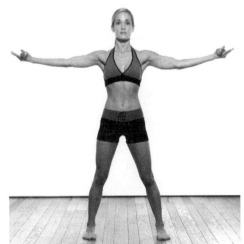

STANDING SHOULDER PRESS

■ Hold your arms extended out to the sides with your elbows bent and forearms reaching for the sky.

■ With weights in hand, face your palms to the front of the room.

■ Lift your arms straight up above your head, straightening your arms as you reach to the ceiling. Do not lock your elbows.

■ Hold your abs in to keep the pressure off your lower back.

■ Return your arms to the starting position.

■ Do 32 reps. This exercise targets your shoulders and back.

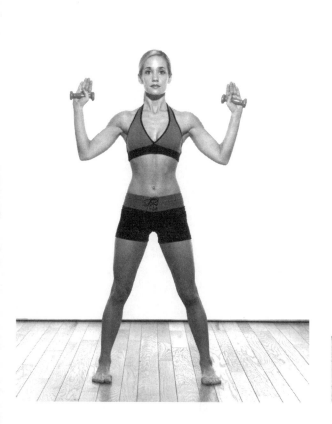
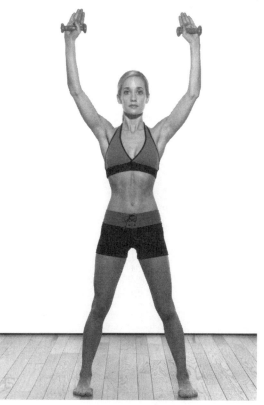

BACK FLY

■ Stand with your feet together, knees slightly bent, torso hinged forward at a 45-degree angle.

■ With weights in hand, hold your arms straight together, dropped down in front of your body. Your palms should be facing each other.

■ Allow your arms to slightly bend and lift them straight out to your sides until they are at shoulder level. As you lift the weights, you want to concentrate on squeezing your shoulder blades together.

■ Do 32 reps. This is a great exercise for building muscle and removing back fat that develops around the bra.

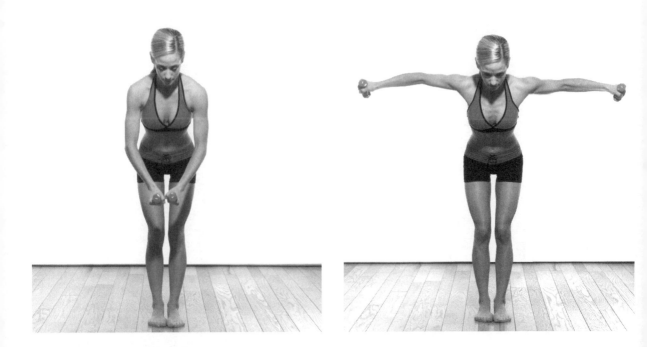

BAY BACK FLY

- Maintain the same standing position—keep your feet together, knees slightly bent, torso hinged forward at a 45-degree angle.

- With weights in hand, hold your arms straight together, dropped down in front of your body. Your palms should be facing each other.

- Leading with your elbows, lift the weights out to your sides.

- Hold in that position.

- From that side position, do small lifts up and down, squeezing in the shoulder blades. This movement is smaller and faster than the bigger Back Fly.

- Do 32 reps.

- Lower your arms back down and return to standing. Remember to always keep your abs in for back support and your chest out.

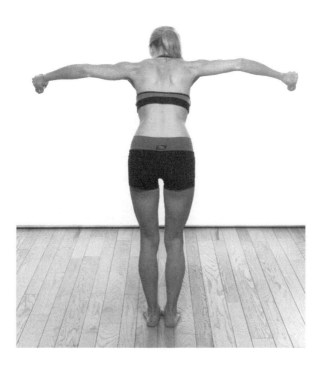

−Stretch−

It's time to slow it down and stretch out the muscles that you just worked. Change the music to something slow and relaxing. Get control of your breath. Breathe full-belly breaths in order to oxygenate your muscles. When stretching, try to hold each pose for approximately 20–30 seconds. Stretches are to be done slowly and fluidly with no sharp or sudden movements. The stretching section should last at least 5 minutes. Take your time and do not underestimate the benefits of a good stretch.

TORSO TWIST STRETCH

■ Lie flat on your back.

■ Bend your right knee and pull your right leg in to your chest.

■ Keep your left leg extended straight on the floor.

■ Cross your right knee over your body to the left, twisting your torso and butt.

■ Keep both shoulders on the floor. This stretch should be coming from your waist.

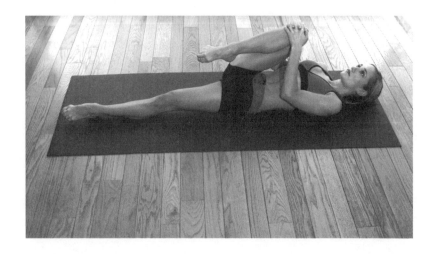

■ If it does not strain your lower back, try to touch your bent right knee to the floor on the left side.

■ Enjoy the stretch in your lower back.

■ Hold this position for as long as you desire.

■ Switch sides and repeat—bending your left knee and keeping your right leg straight along the floor.

■ Cross your left knee over to the right side of your body, touching the floor if you can.

■ Breathe into this stretch, imagining that your breath is going directly to any sore spots, helping to loosen them up.

■ Return your leg to the center of your body.

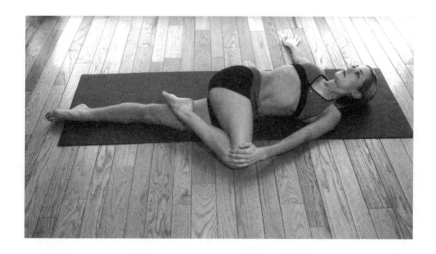

CIRCLES

■ Hug both knees into your chest.

■ Hold your knees with your arms.

■ Make circles with your knees in a clockwise motion, massaging your lower back on the floor.

■ Repeat this motion four times slowly.

■ Return to the center position, hugging your knees into your chest.

■ Reverse directions, making small circles in a counterclockwise motion.

■ Return to the center position, hugging your knees into your chest.

■ Hold this position and breathe into your lower back.

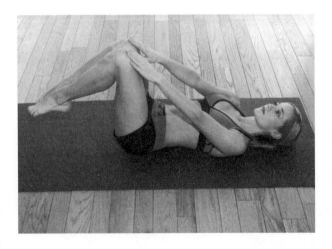
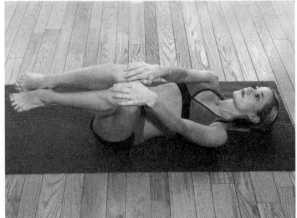

HAMSTRING STRETCH

■ Extend both legs straight out on the floor.

■ Slowly roll up through your back, reaching forward with your fingers.

■ Once in a seated position, continue to stretch your fingers forward, reaching as far as you can. If you can't touch your toes, that is okay. Do not force this stretch. You will feel a slight pull on your hamstrings, but the pull should not be painful.

■ Breathe and hold.

■ Remain in a seated position with your legs stretched out straight.

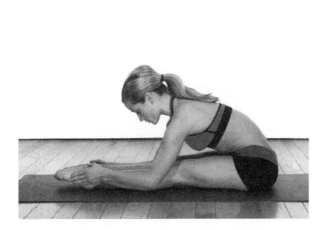
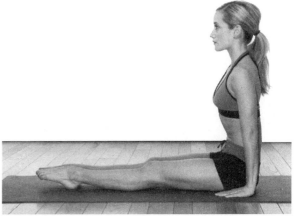

STRADDLED STRETCH

■ Open your legs into a straddle position. Do not bend your knees.

■ Hinge your torso over your left leg and stretch toward your left toes.

■ Hold this stretch for approximately 20 seconds.

■ With your legs still straddled, return your torso to the center position.

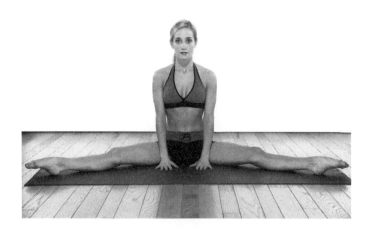

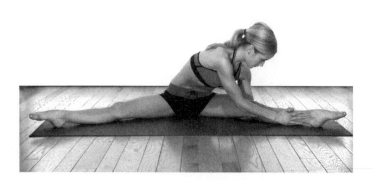

■ Now twist your torso to the right and stretch toward your right toes.

■ Hold this stretch for approximately 20 seconds.

■ Return your torso to center.

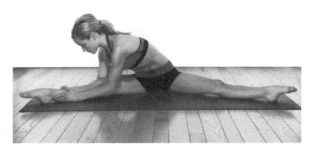

■ Relax your feet and thighs, keep your legs straight, and hinge your body forward between your legs.

■ Try to walk your hands out in front of you. Do not push your muscles to the point of strain. Ease into the stretch. This will stretch your hamstrings and inner thighs.

■ Slowly draw your legs together.

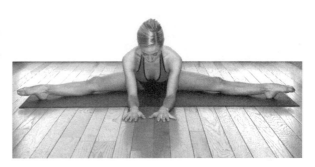

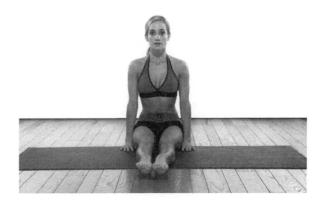

FETAL STRETCH

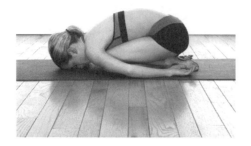

■ Roll over into the fetal position by rolling onto your side (either side). Bend your knees and allow them to fold slightly forward. Rest your head, and all of yourself, on the floor to mentally and physically let go of all tension. This stretch will allow your lower back to relax. It creates space between your spinal cord, allowing your vertebrae to decompress, releasing the pressure that builds up all day.

■ Hold here for 1 minute and just breathe.

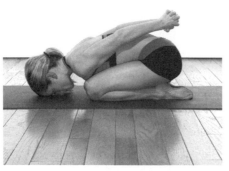

■ While you are still in this position, clasp your fingers behind your back and stretch your arms straight up and over your head. This will lengthen and loosen your shoulders and triceps.

■ Release your arms down, roll onto your back, and bring yourself into a sitting position.

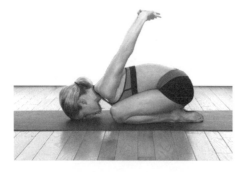

BENT STRETCH

◼ Stand on your feet, but keep your torso hinged over, relaxing your head toward the floor.

◼ Hold for 20 seconds.

◼ Roll up to Standing Position.

◼ Take a deep breath and a gulp of water.

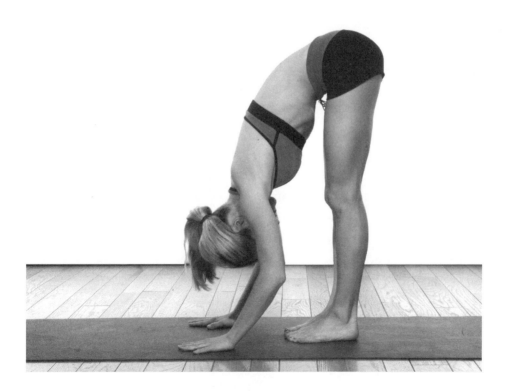

Fit Tip

After a workout, shower at about room temperature. Hot water is relaxing, but it slows circulation and will make you feel sluggish. Cold showers are invigorating but can strain the heart.

Congratulations! You have completed your first Cardio Barre workout! The more you do this program, the better you will get at it. You will increase your strength, flexibility, and endurance.

The moment you tell yourself you can do it . . . you can.

Source of the Sore Muscle

You may remember my telling you in Chapter One that you would be sore after your first workout. You are about to experience what I was referring to. Don't worry, sore muscles are normal. They aren't used to the stress that you are suddenly imposing on them. While soreness undoubtedly hurts, there is a difference between sore and pain. The soreness stems from microscopic rips in the fibers of the connective tissues and muscles caused by your workout (which is a good thing). This microtrauma is a natural and healthy sign of a good workout. The muscles then are filled up with natural waste, like lactic acid, which causes the uncomfortable sensation. Due to this release of lactic and other acids, as well as proteins and hormones, that build up in muscle tissue, you may begin to feel the burn before your workout is even over. The small tears repair themselves, making the muscle grow stronger and harder to tear. The next time you exercise, it will be more difficult to fatigue the muscle to the point of tearing. Don't be alarmed—soreness aches. It might throb, feel stiff, or tight, but as much as it may hurt, it is important to keep your body moving in order to keep the fluids flowing, freeing them from your muscles and relieving the sting.

On the other hand, if you experience sharp, intense, or long-lasting pain, it could mean injury. Injuries are often the result of carelessness. When you are working out, it is important that you pay attention to the movements you are making. How is your alignment? Is your mind wandering? Are you thinking about what you have to do after your workout? Stay in the moment. Stay connected with your body and maintain an awareness of your movements. If something doesn't feel quite right, stop, make an adjustment, or tweak your positioning. If you are in fact injured, you can't exercise it out. The best and fastest way to recover is by resting and healing.

> ## Fit Tip
>
> Try head rolls to relieve muscle ache in your neck and shoulders. Shoulder and arm rolls help release stiffness. Gently walking and doing pliés loosen legs. Stretching and working out will actually help shorten recovery time by eliminating excess fluids in the muscle.

Side-clenching Cramps

When exercising at an optimum level, many may experience cramps. When expelling excess fluids, in other words, when sweating a lot, which you will definitely be doing, muscles can cramp, causing a sensation of intense contractions. Cramps most often occur in the sides, calves, and feet, but can easily be relieved through gentle stretching and often avoided altogether by staying hydrated.

> *If you want the rainbow, you have to put up with the rain.*
> —DOLLY PARTON

Patience

If you feel like your body is on the slow boat to China in terms of seeing change, don't worry, it's totally normal. The first few weeks of a new food and exercise regimen is sure to shock your system and make it question what you are trying to do to it by moving it around so much and denying it of its beloved fat and sugar treats.

Natural High

You have likely heard the term "runner's high." If you haven't, then you have now. A runner's high is a sense of euphoria that is experienced after prolonged cardiovascular exercise. The misconception about a runner's high is that only runners experience it. Not true. The term was coined in the 1970s after appearing in *The Complete Book of Running*. This invincibly happy state is actually a chemical effect caused by the release of endorphins. When bound to receptor points in the brain, they create an analgesic and euphoric sensation. Similar to the effects of opiates, some athletes actually become addicted to this naturally produced chemical, compelling them to continuously push their bodies to the endorphin-discharging threshold. Thought not everyone experiences a "runner's high," exercise is known to alleviate stress and enhance well-being.

BEFORE

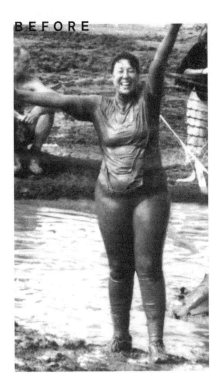

AFTER

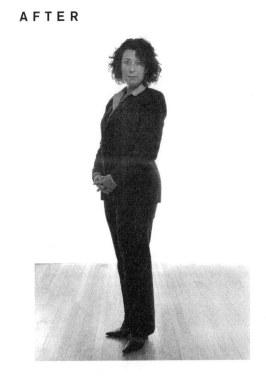

Changed My Life . . .

Deborah Kazenelson Dean, 42, defeated type II diabetes by raising her barre.

Some people are predisposed to have trouble with carbohydrates and the way they affect blood sugar. Once Deborah became pregnant, it was clear that she was one of those people. Before her pregnancy, Deborah was known as having a "naughty body." Not that it was naughty in a bad way, but it was naughty in that it was so good. She had a pretty consistent workout routine from high school through college. Before high school, exercise was not encouraged by her parents. According to Deborah, in the eyes of her South American parents, girls didn't do sports. Those activities were reserved for boys. She never learned to dance—not even ballet or jazz as a little girl—she wasn't on any athletic teams, and she certainly didn't exercise for the sake of bettering her body. Culturally, it was not accepted.

Physical activity was incorporated into her life by accident, or rather, by association. Her best friend was a runner, so Deborah began to run as her running buddy. When she met her husband, she explored his love of skiing, out of the sheer desire to spend more time with him. Because Deborah was easily bored and always looking for a challenge, she began to add additional activities to her repertoire. Hiking with friends added an element of camaraderie and offered extended, uninterrupted talking time. But when she really wanted to workout, she hit the gym. You might have labeled her a "gym rat," since she was regularly seen running any excess calories away on the treadmill. Though running was effective, it was also boring. She never found that "runner's high" that elevates some to a "Zen state." She continued to run, but didn't crave it like others do. To add a little excitement Deborah took a few step classes. Her body stayed tight and "naughty;" that is, until she got pregnant.

Morning sickness became a daily occurrence, to the point that Deborah couldn't keep anything down other than plain, dry bagels and mashed potatoes—of which she consumed a lot of. Soon she had put on 80 pounds and was diagnosed with type II diabetes. Her body unexplainably retained huge amounts of water, which only added to the weight gain. She was tested on a daily basis for preeclampsia. Considering the stellar shape that she had been used to being in, this was a very scary time for her. She was faced with a question—either start taking insulin or make major lifestyle changes and hope they would work. She decided to try the alternative approach—making change. A forward-thinking doctor decided to put her on a high-protein, low-calorie diet to force her body into a state of ketosis—accelerating the speed at which fat stores in her body were burned and used for energy. Her new diet, coupled with a constant exercise program, successfully stabilized her blood sugar levels. Working out became more than a mode to be in great shape, it was suddenly elevated to a much more important level—her health.

Once she delivered her child, she had already begun to get her diabetes under control, but after several tests, doctors found that she had almost no thyroid function. Determined to get her health and her body back without turning to surgery or pills, Deborah's diet continued to consist primarily of protein, while maintaining her exercise program. In time, she was able to balance out her diet, adding salads and some carbohydrates. But, in order to stick to this new lifestyle, she had to find some form of physical activity that wouldn't bore her to the point of losing interest. Running and the occasional step class just wasn't cutting it anymore. She tested the workout waters, from Pilates and yoga to Tae Bo, but nothing seemed to offer enough of a mental or physical challenge. A friend suggested that she try Cardio Barre, and suddenly she found something that aroused both her body and mind!

For Deborah, it was a breath of fresh air to be able to pull any old outfit out of her closet, throw it on, and head to class without feeling like people were expecting an exercise gear fashion show. That's the problem with many gyms; they are often mistaken for pickup joints, requiring you to dress to impress. Working out shouldn't be about putting on a show for anyone else. It should be a very personal time that you devote to yourself, without lurking eyes studying your outfits, checking out your backside, and comparing techniques. It isn't a competition, it isn't about who has better arms or leaner legs, it is about you— only. That is why students keep coming back to Cardio Barre, where all that is important is the dedication of time to yourself.

Coming from a physical activity history of step and running, Deborah found the coordination and grace that came with Cardio Barre elements of exercise that she wasn't used to. Her thighs ached for the first time in a long time—but that was a good thing. What once were squatty calves with odd little bulges poking through, became long and lean. Her waist felt subtly thinner and even her arm muscles slightly stung with the promise of muscular tone. What really took her by surprise was the shrinkage of, what she referred to as, her "Latina tush." She had always viewed her rear end as a big round behind. Suddenly, she realized, it had shrunk slightly, while staying round and strong! With an emphasis on elongating the muscles, in Cardio Barre you avoid easy injuries that short stubby muscles sometimes fall victim to.

While all of Deborah's muscles were gaining strength under her skin, and her pores sweat to the point of exhaustion, the music moved through her, giving her the energy to push through sections of class that were difficult or uncomfortable. It was an interesting dichotomy that she came to embrace—feeling strong and feminine at the same time. Still, as she held her fingers just so, and her toes perfectly pointed, the ballet movements began to feel good to her. Soon, her arm muscles started to gain definition as her stomach became taut. Her tush inched its way up, her thighs gained tone, and that little extra flab of fatty skin over the knees vanished. Her legs were transforming into feminine "dancer's" legs!

Pushing herself and sweating through unfamiliar and sometimes awkward movements, Deborah found that her stamina was more enduring as she became increasingly graceful. Class after class her shoulders crept back and her appearance seemed more poised. And while all of this beauty and grace was taking place, Deborah was shocked at the intensity of each class, an intensity that she was able to keep up with. After a few weeks, she was so proud of the fact that she could sit on a chair with her legs crossed and not feel like she had to hide anything, because there were no longer any dimples or extra flab to conceal! Feeling comfortable in the skin you are in is essential to your self-confidence. Deborah, a public relations consultant, often goes on television on behalf of her clients. If she felt any discomfort or anxiety about her appearance, it would be glaringly obvious to the camera and viewers at home. Instead she exudes strength and grace. So much so that her friends are constantly complimenting her new body and radiating glow. The best is when people you haven't seen for ages approach you and tell you how amazing you look! And, of course, her sons notice that their mom has some seriously toned arms. Sometimes they compare their bicep muscles, flexing to emphasize the definition. And guess who wins those muscle wars?

Deborah depends on her regular 3-times-a-week routine to keep her body tight and her mind sharp. Generally, she gets her workout done in the morning. Though time constraints sometimes cause her to take an evening class, she is a morning person and prefers to get up and out of the house. Getting her workout out of the way first thing leaves her with the rest of the day to not worry about it. Once her workout is done, she goes to work with her eyes wide open and her mind fully awake! Since Deborah has the luxury of working from home, wearing her sweats all day is not out of the ordinary. But when an early morning meeting interferes with her exercise schedule, Deborah simply turns on the TV and does the exercises at home. To make sure she pays equal attention to each side, she repeats each move for the duration of one commercial. After exercising, she plops down at her desk, still sweat soaked, and makes a few phone calls before jumping in the shower. That is when she is very happy that video conferencing hasn't made its way to the mainstream! But, when left as the last thing on her to-do list, the day sometimes gets in the way and her exercise routine falls to the wayside.

More than her morning routine, Cardio Barre has a way of slipping itself into other daily activities. It has been infused into Deborah's daily life, becoming a way of life. Standing stomach exercises have been easily added when talking on the phone, leg lifts make watching TV no longer a stagnant activity. Long lines at the bank lend themselves to subtle calf raises. When doing the dishes Deborah also does squats. She constantly is doing something, as exercise has become a lifestyle.

To occasionally take herself out of her box, and really raise her barre, Deborah does something out of the ordinary every birthday. For her fortieth birthday, she put her body and mind to the test by participating in the Camp Pendleton mud run! More than a challenging 10k race, the mud run is complete with hills, tire obstacles, low sand crawls, river crossings, two 5-foot mud-covered walls that you must scale, a tunnel crawl, slippery hill climb, and the final 30-foot mud pit that you slowly swim or run across. It is an extremely difficult, yet very fun 10k course. Because her stamina was so greatly increased thanks to Cardio Barre, little supplementation was needed to get her in shape for this most challenging task. To prepare, Deborah hired a personal trainer who added weight training to her fitness regimen. She continued doing Cardio Barre 3 times per week—Monday, Wednesday, and Friday, and working with a trainer on her off days. What resulted was a feeling of stretching and condensing, stretching and condensing—stretching from the Cardio Barre, and condensing from the intense weight training. It was a perfect complementary plan for Deborah. Eight thousand people showed up for the mud run. Ironically, Deborah's number was 440 (remember, it was her 40th birthday challenge). After swimming in mud, sliding under tunnels on her stomach, being washed down with fire hoses, and feeling utterly exhausted, two hours later, when she crossed the finish line, Deborah had at least one thousand people behind her! It is one of her biggest accomplishments and sources of pride.

Doing something extreme is certainly exciting, but Cardio Barre is Deborah's constant. It is undoubtedly her workout, but it is also her stress release. When she gets cranky, her kids ask her if she needs to go to the gym. One week without Cardio Barre has a direct effect on her mood. Her work, coupled with two kids and a husband, creates a pretty intense life with a lot of potentially stressful activities going on. When anxiety does creep up on Deborah, her thoughts become compulsive and hyper. To retain control, she comes to class, where she is forced to forget about everything going on outside of her body, because she doesn't have time to contemplate or stress when she is concentrating on keeping up. After her hour, life seems more manageable and her mind calms. With a clear head, she is able to more efficiently tackle challenges, and live in balance. Deborah has actually told me that her biggest fear is that I will get bored of teaching and she will have to find something else to balance her body and mind. (Don't worry—that's not going to happen.)

8

Week Two — Mind Your Body

Congratulations! You have made it through the first week. You finished the hardest part. Living this healthier lifestyle will get easier as we go, and it will become normal for you. It's all about baby steps. We will baby step you all the way to the end of this book, where you will find huge success. So you have proven that you can do Cardio Barre. Don't give up now! You deserve success. You deserve to feel that rush of happiness. You deserve to look in the mirror and smile at the beautiful body that you have sculpted. You deserve to wake up each morning thrilled to experience the day!

There are only two ways to live your life.
One is as though nothing is a miracle.
The other is as if everything is.
—ALBERT EINSTEIN

I know, you may have become comfortable in the skin you were in, comfortable in your life, in your routine, comfortable in comfort. Now is not the time to be comfortable in comfort! Don't settle for mediocrity when you can strive for the best. Don't ever lose sight of the goals that you created for yourself when you were young. The "one day, I am going to be"s, the determination to be the absolute best you can be. Yes, the world is still your oyster! There is life out there, live it! Never lose sight of your goals. Stay determined, positive, and smiling. Take control of your life with every breath. You have set your goal; now keep your mind focused on it. We will make these goals challenging enough to warrant effort, but not too difficult that you will fail. Success breeds success, so we are starting slowly and gradually increasing the effort to watch our progress. Make sure that you acknowledge your progress. Sometimes it is important to step aside and look at the success that you have already achieved. Look at how far you have come. Celebrate your success—the fruit of your labor.

MOVE YOUR BODY: WEEK TWO—3 DAYS, 30 MINUTES

The sections in this second week will include:
Warm-up
Pliés
Torso Twist
Cardio
Upper Body
Stretch

I have designed a specific time frame for you to follow that forces you to develop a workout schedule. In order stay motivated, you must continually challenge yourself—mind and body. You have to work through pain and frustration, work through tears and fleeting thoughts of giving up. Move that body! Burn that fat! Unveil that sexy you from within!

During Week Two we *add* new exercises into the workout that you have already learned in the previous chapter. You will repeat the workout from Week One (page 105) and add one new section—Cardio. The Cardio exercises will directly follow the Torso Twist. So instead of going directly from Torso Twist to Upper Body, we will squeeze in Cardio.

−Cardio−

Your heart is the most important muscle in the body. With exercise, just like any muscle, it will become stronger. Cardiovascular exercise strengthens the heart and lungs. It helps to increase circulation, lift the spirits (thanks to the release of endorphins), and aids in weight loss. If you want to lose weight and slim down, you must do cardio.

Your heart is already pumping hard from the Torso Twist exercises. Now it is time to step it up and increase your body's capacity to burn even more calories. This is not the time to take a lengthy break. If you want a glass of water—fine, but don't let your heart rate dip too low. This section is all about getting that heart rate up! Though the movements within this section might seem like they are separate entities, they are not! Meld them together and let your body flow from one to the next. This section should look like a seamless dance.

STANDING ABDOMINAL EXTENSIONS

■ Stand with your left side angled 45-degrees to the barre.

■ Place your left hand on the barre.

■ Raise your right arm up at an angle into the air.

■ Extend your right leg straight behind you, with your big toe touching the floor.

■ This is your starting position.

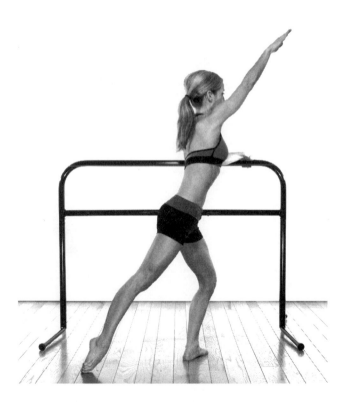

■ Slightly bend your left standing knee.

■ Bend your right knee and bring it up to your chest as you simultaneously pull your right elbow in to meet your knee at your stomach.

■ Return your arm and leg to the starting position. This is not a bouncing motion; rather, it should be smooth and controlled. All of the stress should be placed on the quad muscle, therefore eliminating any stress on the knee joints. The faster you work the harder the heart works.

■ Do 32 reps.

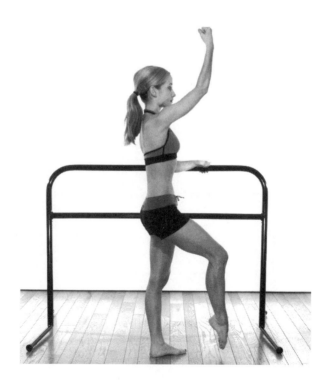

STANDING CRUNCHES

■ Maintaining the same standing position, pull your right knee in to your chest and your right elbow down to meet the knee, but this time, don't return your arm and leg to the original position.

■ This is your starting position.

■ Using your lower abdominals, hold your right knee bent up at chest level and pulse it with small lifts up and down.

■ Simultaneously, pulse your bent right elbow down and up to meet your knee.

■ When lifting your knee, lift it above your waist and lower it below your waist.

■ Repeat this motion 16 times.

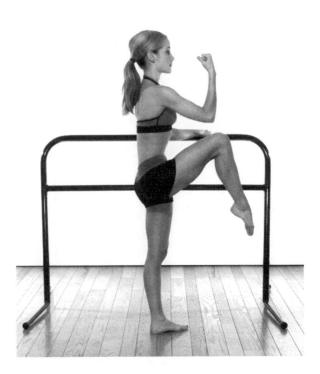

SIDE STANDING CRUNCHES

◼ Stay in the same position as above, but this time, rotate your knee and elbow out to your side.

◼ Again, continually pump your knee and elbow together with small movements. This slight variation on the first pumping exercise targets your obliques (side abdominals).

◼ Do this exercise 16 times.

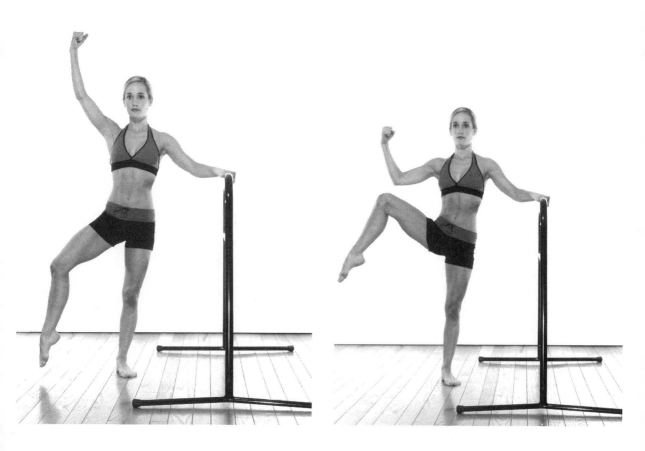

FLAT BACK

■ Stand up straight on a slightly bent left leg and weightlessly rest your right leg beside it.

■ This is your starting position.

■ Hinge your torso forward into Flat Back and extend your right leg out to your side with your right big toe touching the floor.

■ Simultaneously, reach your right arm out to your right side to the height of your shoulder in the motion of a Back Fly (like we did in Warm-up, see page 156).

■ Return both your arm and leg to the starting Standing Position.

■ Repeat for 32 reps.

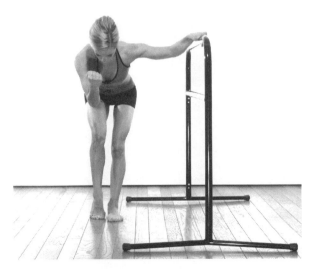
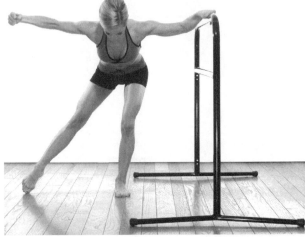

HEEL TOE

■ Stand up straight on a slightly bent left leg and weightlessly rest your right leg beside it.

■ This is your starting position.

■ Extend your right leg forward, and, with a straight leg, tap your heel on the floor in front of you.

■ Simultaneously, press your right arm up toward the ceiling.

■ Return your arm down and your right foot back to the starting position. This is a "heel, toe" movement.

■ Repeat the motion for 32 reps.

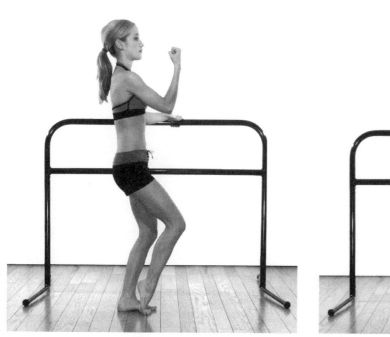
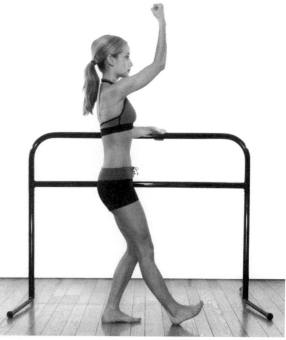

FLAT BACK

■ Return to Flat Back for 16 reps.

LEG EXTENSION—BENT KNEE

■ Stand up straight on your left leg and weightlessly rest your right leg beside it.

■ Lean slightly on the barre.

■ Raise your right leg out to your side until it is at hip level.

■ Bend your right knee and rotate your hip so that your toes are facing up to the the ceiling with a flexed foot.

■ This is your starting position.

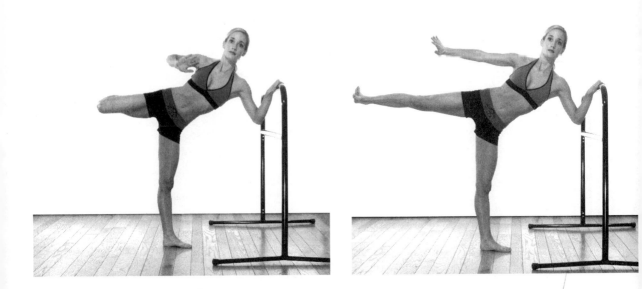

■ Maintain the height of your right leg and press the leg straight out, extending from your body. This is not a kick; it is a press. Squeeze the muscle. It is all about resistance.

■ Simultaneously, press your right arm straight out away from your body parallel to your leg, but at shoulder level.

■ Return to your starting position.

■ Repeat for 16 reps.

LEG EXTENSION—STRAIGHT KNEE

■ Similar to Leg Extension—Bent Knee, hold your right leg out to your side at hip level, but this time, straighten your right leg.

■ Your right foot should be flexed and your toes facing up toward the ceiling.

■ Hold this position for 8 seconds.

■ Lower your leg and repeat the entire series on the other side.

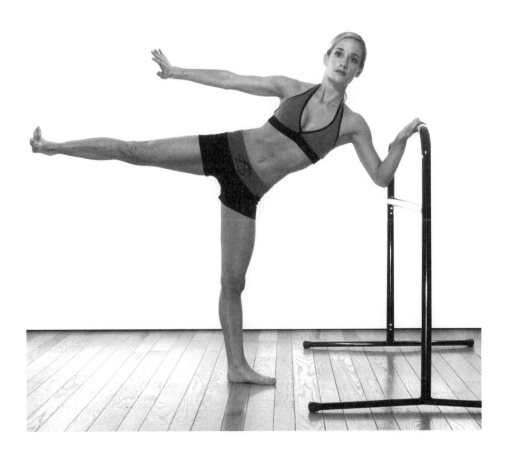

–Other Side–

STANDING ABDOMINAL EXTENSIONS

■ Stand with your right side angled 45-degrees to the barre.

■ Place your right hand on the barre.

■ Raise your left arm up at an angle into the air.

■ Extend your left leg straight behind you, with your big toe touching the floor.

■ This is your starting position.

■ Slightly bend your right standing knee.

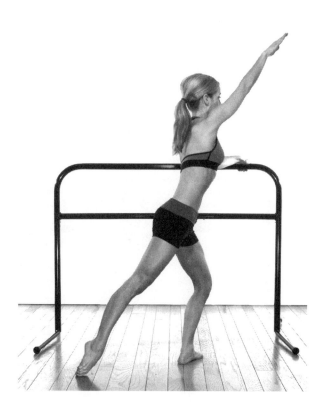

■ Bend your left knee and bring it up to your chest as you simultaneously pull your left elbow in to meet your knee at your stomach.

■ Return your arm and leg to the starting position. This is not a bouncing motion; it should be smooth and controlled. All of the stress should be placed on the quad muscle, therefore eliminating any stress on the knee joints. The faster you work the harder the heart works.

■ Do 32 reps.

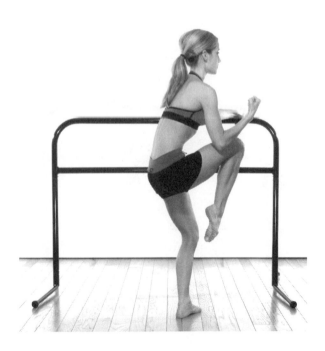

STANDING CRUNCHES

■ Maintaining the same Standing Position, pull your left knee in to your chest and your left arm down to meet the knee, but this time, don't return your arm and leg to the original position.

■ This is your starting position.

■ Using your lower abdominals, hold your left knee bent up at chest level and pulse it with small lifts up and down.

■ Simultaneously, pulse your bent left elbow down and up to meet your knee.

■ When lifting your knee, lift it above your waist and lower it below your waist.

■ Repeat this motion 16 times.

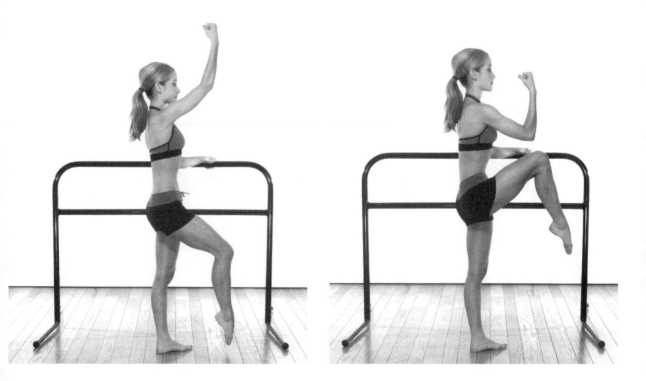

SIDE STANDING CRUNCHES

■ Stay in the same position as above, but this time, rotate your knee and elbow out to your side.

■ Again, continually pump your knee and elbow together with small movements. This slight variation on the first pumping exercise targets your obliques (side abdominals).

■ Do this exercise 16 times.

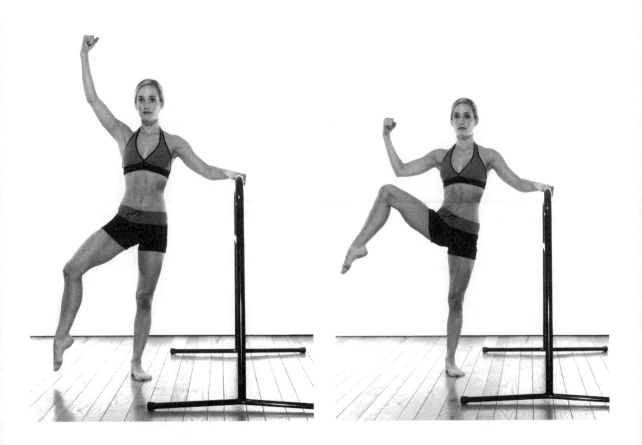

FLAT BACK

- Stand up straight on a slightly bent right leg and weightlessly rest your left leg beside it.

- This is your starting position.

- Hinge your torso forward into Flat Back and extend your left leg out to your side with your left big toe touching the floor.

- Simultaneously, reach your left arm out to your left side to the height of your shoulder in the motion of Back Fly.

- Return both your arm and leg to the starting Standing Position.

- Repeat for 32 reps.

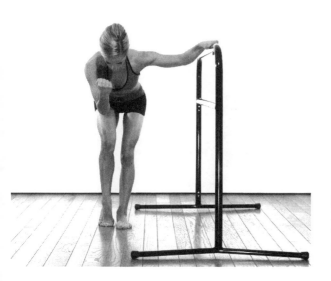
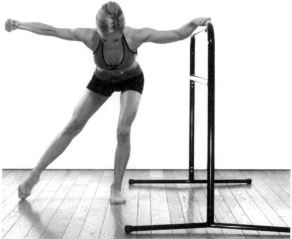

HEEL TOE

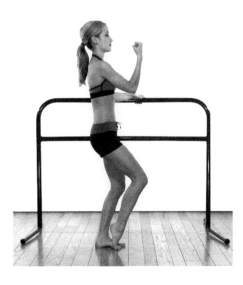

- Stand up straight on a slightly bent right leg and weightlessly rest your left leg beside it.

- This is your starting position.

- Extend your left leg forward, and, with a straight leg, tap your heel on the floor in front of you.

- Simultaneously, press your left arm up toward the ceiling.

- Return your arm down and your left foot back to the starting position. This is a "heel, toe" movement.

- Repeat the motion for 32 reps.

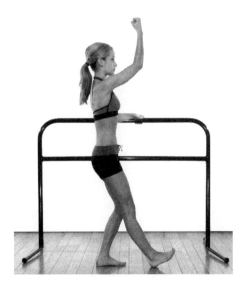

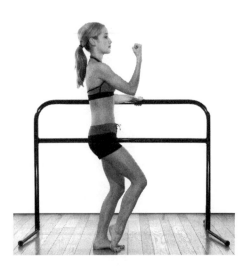

FLAT BACK

◾ Return to Flat Back for 16 reps.

LEG EXTENSION—BENT KNEE

◾ Stand up straight on your right leg and weightlessly rest your left leg beside it.

◾ Lean slightly on the barre.

◾ Raise your left leg out to your side until it is at hip level.

◾ Bend your left knee and rotate your hip so that your toes are facing up to the the ceiling with a flexed foot.

◾ This is your starting position.

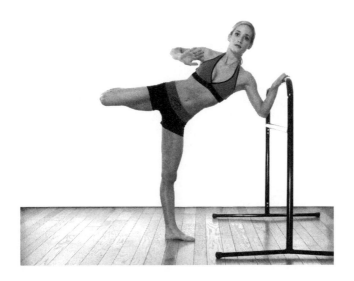

■ Maintain the height of your left leg and press the leg straight out extending from your body. This is not a kick; it is a press. Squeeze the muscle. It is all about resistance.

■ Simultaneously, press your left arm straight out away from your body parallel to your leg, but at shoulder level.

■ Return to your starting position.

■ Repeat for 16 reps.

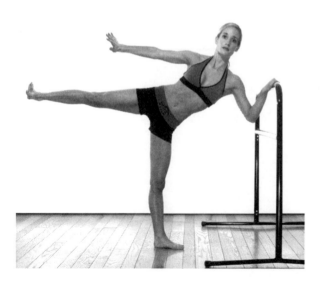
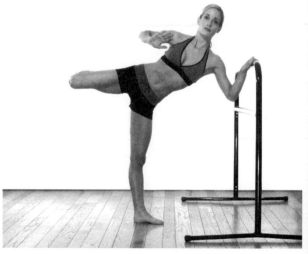

LEG EXTENSION–STRAIGHT KNEE

■ Similar to Leg Extension–Bent Knee, hold your left leg out to your side at hip level, but this time, straighten your left leg.

■ Your left foot should be flexed and your toes facing up toward the ceiling.

■ Hold this position for 8 seconds.

Remember to breathe throughout the exercises. Your muscles need oxygen to work hard, your breath delivers that oxygen. As you gain more balance, stamina, and strength, you will rely less on the barre for support, using your core. Once your cardio endurance improves and you gain more strength and endurance, increase the reps and length of time in this section. If you want to increase your results and burn more fat, do the right side with a weight in your right hand, and do the left side with a weight in your left hand. Work until you sweat.

BEFORE   **AFTER**

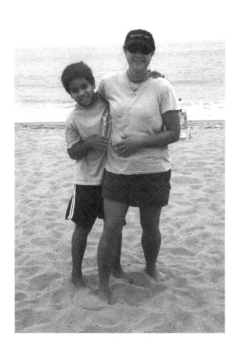
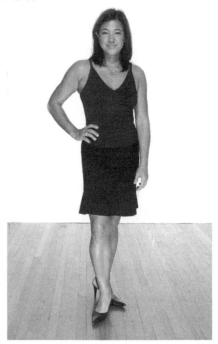

Changed My Life . . .

Scilla Andreen, 42, costume designer and independent film producer, dropped from a size 10 to size 4 and found the courage to leave her husband and follow her passions, all by raising her barre!

Scilla was always told that she was an apple. Well, at least her body was in the shape characteristic of an apple. She compares her body to a boy's, with little definition in the middle. Still, she was pure muscle, especially in her thighs, which tended to bulk. She likes to say that she was "born athletic." As a little girl and through high school she rode crew, downhill skied, ran track, played tennis, sailed, and mountain biked. Dance was definitely not her thing. According to Scilla, she was anything but coordinated. She was an all around outdoorsy girl, constantly active and always in shape. While she was proficient in an array of sports, what she lacked was endurance. She had a hard time with long hauls, but she was great at short spurts. Then she went to college and her athleticism fell to the wayside as partying and smoking won her free time.

When she became pregnant, weight seemed to pile atop her once muscular figure until she gained 65 pounds. She had to have a c-section with both her kids. Her uterus flipped, she had two fibroids and her stomach muscles refused to fuse back together, leaving her with little abdominal strength. The doctors wanted her to have a tummy tuck to get rid of the loose sagging belly skin, but she had so much scar tissue from the keloid and she was afraid of anything invasive. Besides, she had never been a big surgery girl.

She knew she needed to get back in shape, but gyms just weren't her thing. Repeatedly, she found herself joining them with full intention of actually going, but then, a year later, her membership would expire after she had hardly stepped foot past their front doors (except, of course, to purchase the memberships in the first place). Exercise classes never really interested her because she "didn't have that kind of time" or that kind of discipline. Of course, she gave all the classes a shot, testing every emerging trend, like Tae Bo and step, but she felt as though she too quickly mastered them, grew bored, and was ready to move on. Sit-ups, in general, seemed pointless. They required so much daily dedication to wake up, get down on the floor, and do enough to feel a burn—boring! After about a year she finally lost the excess pregnancy weight. Then she decided to challenge herself and train for a marathon. Once she got the breathing down, her endurance levels began to increase, but her body remained the distinct shape of an apple, with little apparent change. Soon, the repetition, again, got monotonous, and Scilla got little joy out of it. On the day of the marathon she blew out both her knees. After she healed up, she attempted to run again, but as soon as she reached the 5-mile marker, her knees throbbed and she had to stop.

In order to cushion her knees while still getting a workout, Scilla tried yoga, but she had no patience for it. She had heard about a no-impact class called Cardio Barre, which happened to be located just down the street from her house. But the idea of a dance-based workout almost instantly turned her away—she was definitely no dancer. Finally, feeling in a bit of a rut (exercise-wise), she decided to buck up and buy a one-class pass. Besides, she was always up for trying something new, that is, until she mastered it. The first class opened her eyes to muscles she never knew she had . . . because they were so sore the morning after! Regardless, to her surprise and with no dance experience to speak of, Scilla could follow the entire class! Of course, the barre was a big help. It created a sense of stability, and offered security. For non-dancers, the fear of losing balance and falling seems to be a common worry. The barre reassures you that you won't fall. Soon, you have your own strength and stability and you no longer need to clasp the barre with your life. But Scilla sure did that first class, and that was okay. And after a very intense sweat session, her knees didn't hurt. Her muscles ached, but I reassured her that that was a good thing, as long as she could walk—which she could.

For the next several classes she maintained her firm grip on the barre, appreciating the security that it offered. In time, her confidence increased and, with the help of her breath, she was able to stabilize her core and avoid toppling over, even when barely holding the barre. Her legs gained flexibility and class after class, they reached a little higher, elongating with each extension. Twelve days later is when she really began to notice change. After class she went home to change for work and, for the first time, her pants hung low on her hips. Nothing fit! Though that was obviously a good thing, in a way she was bummed because she knew that her "fat" clothes, many of which she really liked, were not going to fit her again. She had to invest in an entirely new wardrobe!

Eight weeks later, Scilla swears that her body shape was completely redefined. She came into class so excited that, for the first time in her life, her apple was evolving! With each class, she left a puddle of sweat on the floor as fat and bulky muscle seemingly melted away! Her muscles lengthened, her thighs became long and lean, her calves elongated, her post-pregnancy chest once again found firmness (not that I noticed, that's just what they tell me), muscles replaced any lower back fat, she found that she was actually very flexible and could even do splits, and excess pudge on her stomach melted away as, to the shock of her doctors, her abdominal muscle fibers strengthened and fused together. Without submitting her body to any unnecessary drugs, her cholesterol naturally went down! Scilla no longer considered herself a short-spurt girl as her endurance increased substantially. By strengthening her core, Scilla found that she had incredible balance and better posture. This apple lost her overly muscular, boy-shaped bulk! When before she felt uncomfortable in certain clothes, for fear that her arms might look flabby or her stomach might pooch, now Scilla feels great in anything. Twelve weeks later Scilla struts herself in a size 4!

So, why does someone who hates gyms and gets bored in classes continue to come back? Scilla tells me that she can't master it, that's why she can stick with it. Despite the fact that she labels herself as a tomboy type who prefers outdoor athletics to any sort of dance class, Scilla's stance has changed. After sweating hard for a good hour, she walks out with a distinct gracefulness, her head up, shoulders back, and slightly more elegant. Considering that she has sent about 30 new students my way, I must be doing something right in her eyes! Sometimes friends of hers don't come back again after the first class. They might complain that their backs hurt. But she will ask them if they held their stomach in to protect their back. Of course, the answer is "no." Once they realize that it wasn't the class, but it was them, they are back in, and, after a while, inviting their friends to join them!

Scilla loves the sweating. She once compared herself to the movie *Airplane*, when the pilots were absolutely drenched in sweat sitting in the cockpit. She attributes the sweat to her body's detoxification process. Because, she readily admits, that she likes chocolate and wine, and she sees no sane reason to deprive herself of those rudimentary joys in life. Sometimes, I can tell that she dreads the Cardio part of class. And after she will tell me that she went out the night before, had a few, or maybe four, glasses of wine, and went to bed late. Still, since she has begun taking Cardio Barre, her blood pressure has dropped from high to low, and her cholesterol levels have stabilized.

Because work sometimes gets in the way, Scilla bought a Cardio Barre tape, and, with two taped classes each week, she has stayed in shape. A chair, desk, or kitchen counter take the place of the barre. Sometimes she even uses a doorknob! She keeps it up basically just for maintenance now. Plus, pumping her blood and getting a good stretch feels so good. Some of the exercises have worked themselves into her daily routine, even when that routine has nothing to do with working out! When she is cooking dinner, she might slip in a few leg extensions here and there. Standing in line at the bank or for the restroom at a restaurant, she sometimes does calf raises—going up and down on one toe just enough to make a difference, but hardly enough for anyone to notice.

The physical elements of Cardio Barre, coupled with the fact that it is, according to Scilla, an "un-masterable class," are definitely the main reasons to keep coming, but the mental element plays a big role too. After such an intense workout, these ladies walk out feeling a combination of strong, beautiful, graceful, and powerful. I know, there are some teachers who like to make their students work by screaming at them. That isn't my job. I am not here to yell at you and make you want to make it through a class just to spite me. Do it because it makes you feel so good. Because after a hard class, at the end you really feel like you accomplished something. With that accomplishment, there is a definite sense of empowerment and confidence. Scilla quickly realized that it didn't take much to feel good about herself. As buckets of sweat dripped from her pores, built-up stress released itself from her mind, allowing her thoughts to be crystal clear. With that clarity and increased confidence, she realized that, after eighteen years of marriage to a really nice guy, she wanted a divorce. It wasn't that he was a bad person, but she had a dream and goals, and direction, and he didn't. He wasn't the problem, she was, and it was time for her to leave.

The courage and strength that Cardio Barre gave Scilla, both physically and mentally, helped her get through a divorce. Such a life altering experience, that shakes up what eighteen years of routine has created, requires strength. But, as Scilla learned, that strength has to come from you. Friends and family help, but the majority of your power comes from inside of you. Do you have that power inside of you?

Cardio Barre classes offer Scilla a momentary reprieve, a physical and mental escape from the difficulties of home. An exercise routine offers a safe haven, where you can lose yourself for an hour and emerge into the world with a clear head, while simultaneously doing your body good. Erase the mess in your mind, raise your leg just a little higher, and hold on to that barre! It is empowering on a very personal level.

Scilla came to me the shape of an apple, with high cholesterol, two bad knees, a bad back, and no stomach muscles. She has completely evolved.

9

Week Three — Mind Your Body

Motivation can be hard to come by when results are not yet overwhelmingly apparent. Some of you will be seeing results by now, and others may not yet. Stay with it. Your body is changing from the inside, and sometimes it takes a little while to push through to the outside. But believe me, change will happen very soon. Don't limit your success by giving up on yourself and on me. In fact, let's eliminate the word "limitation" from your vocabulary. Your bodies and minds are limitless and you can achieve anything you want . . . if you set a goal, believe you can do it, and focus—success is sure to follow.

I don't care what cards you were dealt in life, you all deserve to have everything you desire, everything you strive for, everything you dream and fantasize about. Oftentimes the biggest hindrance to achieving the most that you can from life is yourself. That's right. You go around putting yourself down, blaming others for your failures and misfortunes, and making yourself believe that you can't. Guess what, when you tell yourself "I can't" enough, then you can't. Good job, you have actually convinced yourself that you cannot be any better than you are, that you don't deserve any more than you have, that you won't achieve all of the happiness that those around you get to experience. No! Erase any and all of those negative thoughts from your mind. Pretty soon, those "I can't" thoughts become mantras. Promise me this, from now on, whenever one of those "I can't" mantras enters your mind, bulldoze them down with "Yes I can!"

All you need to do is welcome positive change. No matter where we are in life, or how successful we are, we can always improve, better ourselves, or grow from that level of existence. You have to believe and know that there is always more . . . because there is! I am talking about positive growth. Your body is where all of your thoughts, dreams, and purpose are stored. Take care of it and honor it and it will take care of you. It will be the vehicle to operate at peak performance.

All great achievers in life did not just have an aimless goal, they had a definite goal, and they believed in their ability to achieve it, and they did. Lance Armstrong could not have won those races if he didn't believe, without a doubt, that he could do it. Despite the doctors telling him that he would never race again, he went out and won more races than anyone . . . ever! You do deserve happiness, you can achieve success. And, you know what, with that attitude you will!

Excuses don't make the body, action does. Keep your body moving!

Difficulties are meant to rouse,
not discourage. The human spirit is
to grow strong by conflict.
—WILLIAM ELLERY CHANNING

MOVE YOUR BODY: WEEK THREE—4 DAYS, 30 MINUTES

The sections in this third week will include:
Warm-up
Pliés
Torso Twist

Cardio
Upper Body
Stretch

Fit Tip

After a workout, it is important that you shower within 1 hour. You want to wash away the toxin-filled sweat that coats your skin.

You have made it this far, and you are doing great! Those first two weeks are the hardest. You are breaking old habits and creating new healthier ones. Most of the aches and pains should be lessening now, and you should be feeling a little stronger and leaner.

It is time to begin to hone in and up the ante. We are sticking to the same program as last week, but we are adding another day. Hone in on your intentions and increase your intensity to help maintain your enthusiasm and see your goal.

You are ready to add one more workout day to your week. Pick a day that fits into your schedule, but try and keep Sundays off. This week, your routine will consist of the same exercises, in the same order for the same amount of time; you are simply adding one extra day. The more you exercise the stronger and leaner you will get, the better you will feel, and the more your body will crave it on a daily basis.

To keep your interest, surround yourself with things that motivate you. Maybe place an old picture of yourself at your worst at the foot of your bed or on the refrigerator to make you want to strive even harder to get as far away from that old you as possible. Or, on the other hand, put up a photo of you at your best, or a photo of a celebrity who has your ideal body to remind you of your goals and where you one day want to be. Put either image where you will see it daily.

Many of you might feel motivated by seeing yourselves in new slim clothes. If you like to shop—go out and buy one fabulous outfit to celebrate your success so far. Get something that makes you feel sexy, because you are!

Of course, the road to success is not always straight and spotless. It is normal for you to encounter a few setbacks. But stay strong! You will have both successes and failures, but you must focus on the successes, not dwell on the failures.

BEFORE **AFTER**

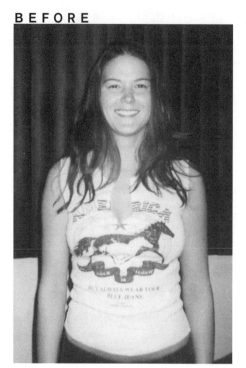
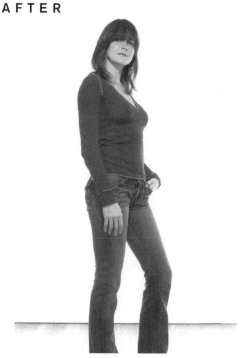

Changed My Life . . .

Elizabeth Devin, 31—Cardio Barre helped Elizabeth kick a 14-year alcohol addiction and proved that you can get high on life!

Some students find that exercise becomes almost an addiction—a healthy one. Elizabeth turned to Cardio Barre to help her to get over an unhealthy one—alcohol. She had been living in Florida as a bartender, a party girl and, for fourteen years, an alcoholic. The booze helped her forget about her troubles, allowing her to live in her own fantasyland . . . for a time. Then it stopped working and it began to act exactly as it is—a depressant. The fun part that made her feel light on her feet and high in her head turned to heaviness and sadness. Life was no longer a party. When Elizabeth made the move to Los Angeles, a friend decided to show her the town and introduce her to her new life. She was even introduced to Cardio Barre. But Elizabeth took one look at the rows of women sweating up a storm and thought we were all crazy! She finally decided to surrender herself, and she went to AA, beginning her path to sobriety.

In need of a healthy activity to fill the void that was once flooded by alcohol, Elizabeth thought back to that crazy class filled with sweaty women and decided to give it another shot. She loved it! Of course, not having exercised much in her life, the class was definitely a challenge. She stood in the back corner of the room, barely making it through to the end. Everything was a challenge for her—the leg lifts were a struggle, she could hardly lift the weights during arm work, the stomach exercises were stingingly painful. By the end of class, her body made it brutally clear just how unhealthy and out of shape she was. Still, she subconsciously knew that this class would be very good for her . . . and she came back the next day. Her muscles were really sore for a long time. Even going to the bathroom was painful because it forced her to sit down. But for some reason she liked that feeling. It made her aware of her body. As they say, pain is a bridge to change. Elizabeth's addictive personality made her need more. So she quickly became a regular student. After a few classes, her face broke out in toxin releasing pimples, an experience that was humbling for Elizabeth.

Elizabeth essentially traded one addiction for another, but this time the drug was her body. She would arrive 30 minutes early to stretch and stay 30 minutes after to cool down. Whenever I motivated the class by reminding them that success is 70 percent mental and you can do anything you want if you can put your mind to it, her eyes lit up. In a matter of weeks, Elizabeth's body had already dramatically changed. After 3 months she had "six-pack" abs and sculpted arms. She was strong and lean everywhere. The alcohol-induced puffiness and bloat deflated. Her muscles became toned, her legs had definition, and her butt lifted about 2 inches! Now her friends call her their "fitness guru." She has become an inspiration, a testament to the benefits of exercise and health. Ironic considering the intentional devastation that she put her body through on a daily basis for so many years. In hopes of achieving such startling success, a few friends have dabbled in Cardio Barre themselves. In fact, one of them lost 20 pounds in 1 month!

More than revealing a really incredible body that had been concealed under several layers of puffiness, Elizabeth came to understand that the alcoholism had masked her problems, hiding her fears. Cardio Barre taught her to let go of them, completely release them from her life so that they could no longer torment her. Sometimes she would cry after class. But her tears were not out of sadness; instead they represented her total surrender. It was as though a stream of pent-up emotions that had been locked up in her body were finally being let go and liberated! Toxins raced from her pores, leaving her a bit dizzy from the deep cleanse, but lighter in both spirit and body. The endorphins gave her a much better high than any other drug that she had tried. That in itself was a feat for Elizabeth—to realize that she could get high from life and was no longer a slave to alcohol for happiness.

Life now has new meaning to Elizabeth. It matters now. Whereas her body used to be the recipient of years of abuse, health now matters to her. Spiritual well-being now matters to her. Cardio Barre has become an essential element of Elizabeth's sanity-saving routine. She goes to AA meetings three times per week, and Cardio Barre four times per week. To her, it is more than a workout for her body, it is where she actually goes to work out issues, problems, doubts, and frustrations. It is where she unties mind and body, only leaving class each day when she feels completely whole.

Now, whenever she doesn't do Cardio Barre, Elizabeth is noticeably crabby, edgy, and sensitive. Cardio Barre helps Elizabeth just be healthy and in the moment. It has become a tool that helps her to dig up and throw out disease instead of concealing it in alcohol and pretending it isn't there.

To further improve the state of her body, Elizabeth has altered her diet. She used to pretty much eat whatever she was in the mood for. Not anymore. Since becoming sober, her body is experiencing a heightened sensitivity to sugar. Just a little will make her jittery and unnaturally high. Obviously, alcohol and drugs are out of the question. Elizabeth was looking to do more than change her body, she was determined to change her life.

10

Week Four — Mind Your Body

Once you complete this week, you will have successfully finished your first month! Do you know how huge this is? HUGE! Congratulations!

How are you feeling? What is going on in your body? Take time to take note. Do a full body scan. Close your eyes and put all of your focus on your toes. Now slowly move your attention up to your ankles, calves, knees, thighs, butt, hips, waist, bust, shoulders, neck, face, and finally your head.

Anything going on that I should know about? Do you feel any soreness? Do you feel tighter? Stronger? Leaner? Less flabby? How do your clothes fit? Are your jeans a little less snug? What about your "tester skirt?" How's it fitting? Well, guess what? You look gorgeous. You do!

Look at yourself in the mirror. Appreciate the changes, no matter how big or how small they might be. If you have truly stuck it out, and diligently stayed with the program, the changes in your body and attitude should be dramatic by weeks end. Feel inspired by your own achievements and surround yourself with people who have positive attitudes toward success, especially yours!

It takes about a month for your body to break old habits and adjust to the new ones. In a few days, your first month is up! Old habits broken! New habits here we come! Reward yourself for your successes. Your reward could be a new outfit, a special dinner out, or a weekend away for a little relaxation. Believe me, you deserve it. I know how hard you have worked. You should be proud of yourself. I am!

MOVE YOUR BODY: WEEK FOUR—4 DAYS, 40 MINUTES

The sections in this fourth week will include:
Warm-up
Pliés
Torso Twist
Cardio
Barre Thighs
Upper Body
Stretch

It is time to take your workout a step further. Why do many of you tout the ballet body as the best body? It's all about the legs! This week I am introducing a section that will specifically target your thighs! At the end of this section, you will feel the burn, but that is definitely a good thing. It takes a lot to change the legs, considering that they already carry the burden of you all day. Think about it: your legs are constantly working out. Whenever you walk around, they are carrying you. Whenever you sit or stand, they lift and lower you. Not only are they moving, expanding, and contracting, but they are carrying your body weight! If you want to change your legs, you are really going to have to stress them out and make them work like they never have before. Are you ready? Let's do this!

You will repeat the workout from Week Three, but this week I am adding one new section: Barre Thighs. You will add Barre Thighs directly after Cardio. If you feel the need to take a breather before we begin, fine. But don't rest for too long. Take a few sips of water, catch your breath, and let's do this!

−Barre Thighs−

OUTER THIGH LIFT

■ Face the barre and stand up straight.

■ Now, with your tummy pulled up, spine straight, and head in line with your spine, hinge your torso forward so that it is parallel to the floor—like a table. Your torso is at a complete 90-degree angle and your legs are perpendicular to the floor. In order to maintain Flat Back, your core is activated and your hamstrings are elongated.

■ Place your hands loosely on the barre in front of you. Your arms should be straight, but keep your elbows soft (not bent, but not locked either). The barre is not there to hold all of your weight; it is there as a safety net to help you maintain your balance until your core is strong enough to take over.

■ Your left leg will begin as your supporting leg.

■ Bend your right knee, but keep your knees together.

■ Point the toes on your right foot.

■ This is your starting position.

■ Maintaining Flat Back position, lift your right knee out to the side until it reaches hip level. You will keep your right knee bent and aligned with your left knee. Keep you toes pointed.

■ Lower your right knee back down to your left knee, but keep your knee bent. Your right toes should not touch the floor for the duration of this exercise. This is an isolation exercise of the outer thigh. By working one muscle group at a time, you will isolate and sculpt one body part at a time. Lift your knee up and down in a controlled motion. Be sure that you keep your abs in, in order to support your lower back.

■ Repeat for 32 reps.

SCORPION LEG LIFT

■ Maintain Flat Back position with your hands loosely placed on the barre, left leg supporting and right knee bent. But this time, you will lift your right leg behind you, while maintaining a semi-bent knee. Your right knee should be directly behind your butt. Turn your leg out slightly so that your outer thigh is facing up toward the ceiling. Imagine that your leg is a scorpion's stinger curving up behind your body. During this exercise, you will be trying to sting your own head.

■ This is your starting position.

■ Lift your right leg up. Since the starting position of your knee is butt level, try to lift your knee a few inches above your butt. The weight of your leg is your resistance, sculpting your thighs. By keeping your leg turned out, you will stretch the quad muscle while sculpting the outer thigh.

■ Return to your starting position.

■ Lift and down for 16 reps.

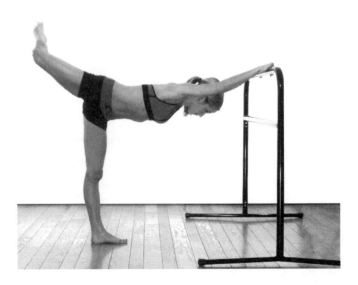

SCULPTING LEG EXTENSIONS

■ Maintain Flat Back position with your hands loosely placed on the barre, left leg supporting and right knee bent. But this time, lift your right knee out to your side at hip level. Point your toes to the back right corner of the room. Rotate your leg out so that your outer thigh is facing upward.

■ This is your starting position.

■ Extend your right leg straight out, pressing it to the right corner of the room. Your knee should stay is the starting position; it is only the bottom half of your leg that extends out. The knee does not move.

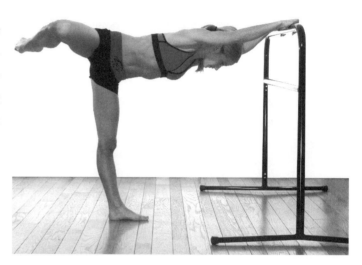

■ Return your leg to the starting position.

■ Repeat this leg extension for 16 reps.

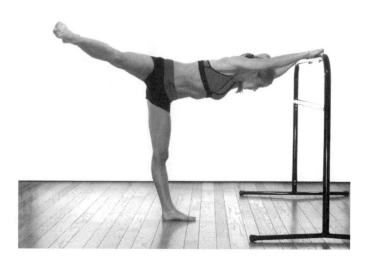

ANGLED LEG EXTENSIONS

■ Maintain Flat Back position with your hands loosely placed on the barre, left leg supporting and right knee bent. Extend your right leg out to the back right side corner of the room (this is the second position of Sculpting Leg Extensions). Turn your right outer thigh out so that it is facing the ceiling (the muscle group that is facing up is the one that is working). Point your toes. Both legs should be straight.

■ This is your starting position.

■ Do small leg lifts up and down. Since your right leg is at hip level for your starting position, be sure to raise it a few inches above hip level for each lift.

■ Do 16 reps.

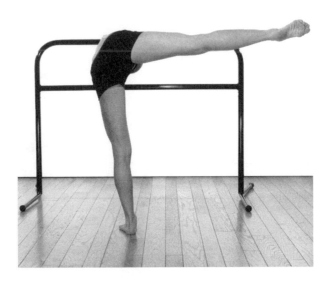

LEG EXTENSIONS

■ Maintain Flat Back position with your hands loosely placed on the barre. This time, extend your right leg directly behind you to the back of the room. Point your toes. Both legs should be straight.

■ This is your starting position.

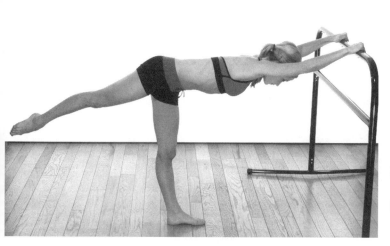

■ Do small lifts up and down. Since your leg is extended at hip level for your starting position, try to lift it a few inches above hip level.

■ Do 16 reps.

■ Hold your leg up for 8 seconds and lower down to standing position.

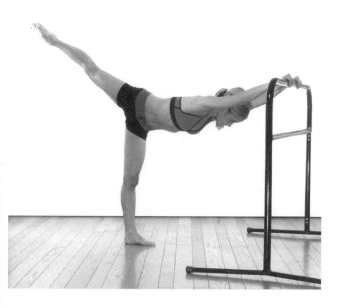

STRETCH

■ Keep your legs straight, but hinge your torso over, flopping down to reach your toes. This position stretches out your back muscles and relieves tension. It is a great stretch to do any time.

■ Stand up and repeat the other side.

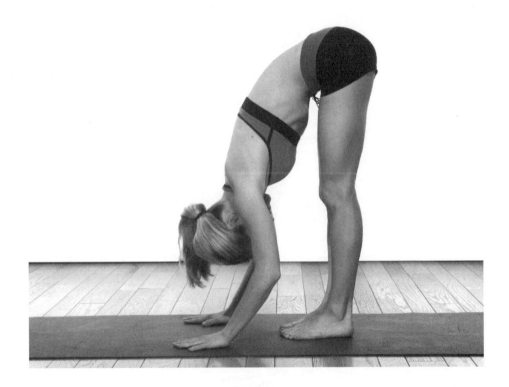

−Other Side−

OUTER THIGH LIFT

■ Face the barre and stand up straight.

■ Now, with your tummy pulled up, spine straight and head in line with your spine, hinge your torso forward so that it is parallel to the floor—like a table. Your torso is at a complete 90-degree angle and your legs are perpendicular to the floor. In order to maintain Flat Back, your core is activated and your hamstrings are elongated.

■ Place your hands loosely on the barre in front of you. Your arms should be straight, but keep your elbows soft (not bent, but not locked either). The barre is not there to hold all of your weight; it is there as a safety net to help you maintain your balance until your core is strong enough to take over.

■ Your right leg will begin as your supporting leg.

■ Bend your left knee, but keep your knees together.

■ Point the toes on your left foot.

■ This is your starting position.

■ Maintaining Flat Back position, lift your left knee out the side until it reaches hip level. You will keep your left knee bent and aligned with your right knee. Keep you toes pointed.

■ Lower your left knee back down to your right knee, but keep your knee bent. Your left toes should not touch the floor for the duration of this exercise. This is an isolation exercise of the outer thigh. By working one muscle group at a time, you will isolate and sculpt one body part at a time. Lift your knee up and down in a controlled motion. Be sure that you keep your abs in, in order to support your lower back.

■ Repeat for 32 reps.

SCORPION LEG LIFT

■ Maintain Flat Back position with your hands loosely placed on the barre, right leg supporting and left knee bent. But this time, you will lift your left leg behind you, while maintaining a semi-bent knee. Your left knee should be directly behind your butt. Turn your leg out slightly so that your outer thigh is facing up toward the ceiling. Imagine that your leg is a scorpion's stinger curving up behind your body. During this exercise, you will be trying to sting your own head.

■ This is your starting position.

■ Lift your left leg up. Since the starting position of your knee is butt level, try to lift your knee a few inches above your butt. The weight of your leg is your resistance, sculpting your thighs. By keeping your leg turned out, you will stretch the quad muscle while sculpting the outer thigh.

■ Return to your starting position.

■ Lift and down for 16 reps.

SCULPTING LEG EXTENSIONS

■ Maintain Flat Back position with your hands loosely placed on the barre, right leg supporting and left knee bent. But this time, lift your left knee out to your side at hip level. Point your toes to the back left corner of the room. Rotate your leg out so that your outer thigh is facing upward.

■ This is your starting position.

■ Extend your left leg straight out, pressing it to the left corner of the room. Your knee should stay is the starting position; it is only the bottom half of your leg that extends out. The knee does not move.

■ Return your leg to the starting position.

■ Repeat this leg extension for 16 reps.

ANGLED LEG EXTENSIONS

■ Maintain your flat back position with your hands loosely placed on the barre, right leg supporting and left knee bent. Extend your left leg out to the back left side corner of the room (this is the second position of Sculpting Leg Extensions). Turn your left outer thigh out so that it is facing the ceiling (the muscle group that is facing up is the one that is working). Point your toes. Both legs should be straight.

■ This is your starting position.

■ Do small leg lifts up and down. Since your left leg is at hip level for your starting position, be sure to raise it a few inches above hip level for each lift.

■ Do 16 reps.

LEG EXTENSIONS

■ Maintain Flat Back position with your hands loosely placed on the barre. This time, extend your left leg directly behind you to the back of the room. Point your toes. Both legs should be straight.

■ This is your starting position.

■ Do small lifts up and down. Since your leg is extended at hip level for your starting position, try to lift it a few inches above hip level.

■ Do 16 reps.

■ Hold your leg up for 8 seconds and lower down to standing position.

Fit Tip

You MUST keep your abs pulled in for back support. If you feel tension in your back it is because of weak back muscles and improper alignment. As you get stronger and as your technique and placement improve, your back will experience less tension. Be sure to support your back with your abs in order to avoid injury.

STRETCH

- Keep your legs straight, but hinge your torso over, flopping down to reach your toes. This position stretches out your back muscles and relieves tension. It is a great stretch to do anytime.

- Barre Thighs are Cardio Barre signature moves, and they are extremely effective in shaping your hips, butt, and thighs. Placement is very important, and it will take some time to master it completely. Patience and focus will get you there. The secret is learning to use your abs for body support and not relying on the barre. Be aware of your placement with all body parts at all times. Proper posture is a must. Work at a steady and fluid pace throughout the exercise, but do not rush. Once you feel comfortable with the movements and are ready for a challenge, add additional reps.

BEFORE **AFTER**

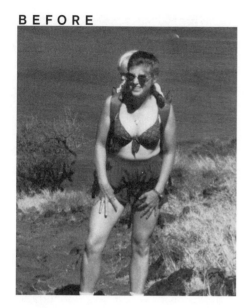
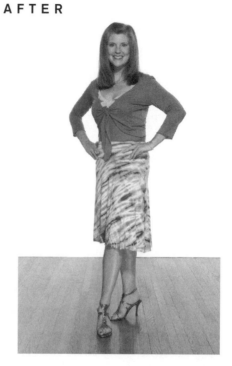

Changed My Life . . .

Joan Hardie, 42, found calm within chaos through Cardio Barre.

Joan has always realized the benefits of exercise. As a nurse, constantly caring for patients who are recuperating after surgery, she sees the real benefits of physical activity—life. Regardless of age, Joan notices a huge disparity between patients who are in shape, and those who are not. By and large, patients who are in shape heal faster than those who aren't. The really physically fit people bounce back so quickly that they are ready to leave the hospital before the doctor writes the discharge order. On the other hand, people who are overweight and don't exercise tend to max out their time in the hospital—not that they are doing it intentionally, but it is so much harder for them to get out of bed and move around after surgery. More than physically healing, Joan notices that healthy people are more motivated and compliant. They are physically and emotionally determined to get well.

To maintain the health of her own body, fitness has been a constant in Joan's life. But, like many of my students, she always looked for alternatives to the typical gym experience. Still, sometimes the convenience of the gym seems unbeatable, so she bought a membership. Preferring group exercise classes to working out on equipment, Joan depended on the numerous class offerings held at the gym. She sampled step and aerobics classes but, while sometimes the classes were great, they more often were not. The problem was a lack of consistency. You never knew which teacher was going to lead each class, creating a constant variance in teaching style, structure, and level. Preferring not to leave her exercise classes up to chance, Joan began taking ballet classes twice a week. She loves the refinement of ballet, the beauty in the movements, the stretch and the balance.

Joan discovered Cardio Barre while flipping through the *Los Angeles Times*. Intrigued by the cardio/dance combo, and in search of a fun and dependable class that would help her lose weight and get in shape, she came to a class. The first class, in her words, "kicked my butt!" Considering that she took twice-weekly ballet classes coupled with cardio classes twice a week, she was shocked to find herself panting halfway through class, gasping for air and taking frequent breaks. Her face was beet red, and she was pouring sweat. The next morning, her intensely sore body reminded her of the concentrated workout she had put herself through the morning before. She knew that she had finally found her perfect workout—combining heart-pumping exercise that made her work up a major sweat, along with the grace and body awareness of dance. Of course, what creates a sweat is working your butt off, which, sometimes, is painful. But with most healthy change comes a bit of pain. Thankfully, the music helped Joan get through the really challenging moves, giving her something else to think about and focus on.

Significant weight loss was not the first physical sign that Cardio Barre was working for Joan. It was muscle tone. Her body seemed to lean and lengthen, as muscles became increasingly defined. Soon, her metabolism kicked in and her body began to process and burn foods and fat more efficiently. Her body was molding into her perfect body!

Ballet remains a constant in Joan's life, but taking Cardio Barre several times each week has significantly improved her endurance and strength. Other ladies in ballet often comment on the weight she has lost and the transformation of her now lean, firm, and toned body. As her body slims down to a svelte size, stress is eased from her mind, which is definitely essential for a woman working 12-hour shifts four days a week in a hospital filled with injury and illness! Nurses don't have the option of "getting to that later," when duty calls they have to be there. No procrastinating, no exceptions. It is the type of job that makes you feel like you are never doing enough. The constant deadlines—from minute to major—keep nurses relentlessly running around with a slew of things to do within the next ten minutes! From blood draws and blood sugar checks to simply asking how a patient is doing, Joan is constantly checking the clock to make sure that she is on top of all the little details, completing all of the orders that doctors write, talking with family members, taking care of the patients, going, going, going! It is physically and mentally exhausting!

To decompress, a lot of nurses turn to food—comfort food, which only aggravates the problem. Similar to depending on alcohol for comfort, depending on food only makes you feel worse in the long run. They may bring some solace for a few seconds, but, at the end of the day, all you have done is numb the pain, not made it go away. Alcohol gives you a headache the next morning, and food adds several inches to your waistline. Joan avoids such self-destructive behavior by turning to exercise to cleanse frustrations from her system. After a long day at work, the last thing that Joan can muster is enough energy to take a rigorous Cardio Barre class, so instead she takes class in the mornings on her off days. Exercising the morning after a 12-hour shift helps wipe her slate clean of any residual frustration or stress that may linger from her job. She sweats away toxic energy and negative emotions, refreshing her mind and spirit, and allowing her to be fully present, effective, and on her toes. Stress is unlikely to upset her or wane on her patience, allowing her to tend to doctors, patients, and the families of patients. Working out first thing in the morning also gives her a burst of energy that lasts throughout the day.

Of course, sometimes Joan does go out a little later than she should the night before, and her body makes its resentment very clear, providing little energy to complete class. It is amazing how you can gauge the health of your body through exercise. When you neglect to give it enough rest, when you fill it with unhealthy foods, or when you indulge in a few too many drinks, your body revolts by withholding precious energy, essential to an effective workout and maintaining energy throughout the day.

Because Cardio Barre has become such an important element to Joan's life, she has begun to minimize activities that impede her energy and take from her "me-time." Joan depends on her one hour of Cardio Barre to replenish her energy and her spirit. It is her time to work on herself. Cardio Barre requires that you pay attention to your coordination. Rarely does a routine become rote like running. It is more than merely one foot in front of the other. You are forced to put both your mind and body into the work, which minimizes distractions and wandering thoughts. That fight with your husband, breakup with your boyfriend, misunderstanding with your friend, feelings of insecurity, embarrassment or anger, are all checked at the door. Once those endorphins start flowing, life is beautiful, and so are you! That is the reason that Joan keeps coming back—the endorphin release, the runner's-high buzz, the feeling that today is going to be a very good day! You rarely just stand there staring at yourself in the mirror and critiquing your body. Occasionally, it might take a little longer to focus your mind and get into your body, but once it clicks you feel . . . alive, invigorated, completely connected!

11

Week Five — Mind Your Body

If you remained committed, you have broken your bad habits. Your body is suddenly drastically evolving, as though after all of your hard work, it finally clicked. Pounds are shedding from your body as your svelte figure is emerging. It is working! Your attitude is adjusting. You are beginning to view fitness as a way of life, no longer a chore. One month gone, one month to go. The rest of your life is just upkeep and enjoying this new body that you have sculpted. You have already accomplished so much. And you know that. So does everyone around you. You are beginning to glow, which is one of the most beautiful qualities in a woman.

Now that you have shed so many emotional and physical pounds, it is natural to want to eat healthier and take care of yourself. You will become addicted to this lifestyle, and it is a great and healthy addiction. So, this book truly is about "raising your bar" in life and taking yourself to the next level. Allow yourself to move up to the next level. You deserve it. Be the best you that you can be. Don't let anyone, including yourself, sabotage your success. Put yourself and your happiness first. I know it can be hard, especially if you are used to constantly doing for everyone else. But this is your time to shine, it is your time to take center stage, take it with all you've got!

No matter how successful you are or how challenged you are, your life can always be better than it is. So when you are ready to make a change, you must raise your standards. Considering that you have already come so far, you are clearly ready to make change. If you have the courage to claim it, the world is yours, and the first step is about changing yourself. But you must believe. Empowering your beliefs is behind great success.

You must set a standard for yourself or you will fall back to old unhealthy patterns. Being interested in a goal and committing to it are two very different concepts. Commitment, dedication, and purpose will lead you to success. Don't make excuses for failure. Zero in on your goals and they will be fulfilled. Having a plan will help you make quality decisions along the way. Just as muscles get stronger as we use them, so does the mind while making decisions. Flex your mental muscles. You are strong, both inside and out.

MOVE YOUR BODY: WEEK FIVE–5 DAYS, 40 MINUTES

The sections in this fifth week will include:
Warm-up
Pliés
Torso Twist
Cardio
Upper Body
Stretch

Wow! We are about to begin the second half of your road to success. You are now ready to take the horse by the reins and ride! Your body is chemically changing. It feels good when it works out, and bad if you miss a few days. You have to get up and work out, or else you are tired. But just because you are losing weight and looking good, does not mean that it is time to slack. You have to continue to push yourself. You are your priority. If you don't take the time and make the room to change your body, no one else will. Excuses don't work here. You do.

We will step up the workouts to 5 days this week. You will repeat the same routine from Week Four, you will just add one extra day. I know, 5 days a week sounds like a lot, but you can fit it in. Think about the 40 minutes here and there that you waste watching television, lounging around, fiddling through busy work, and being a chatty Cathy kibitzing with your girlfriends. You can make better use of your time by dedicating it to your body. Stay strong and focused. If you feel that you need a little extra motivation, talk to others about your goals. Vocalizing your goals makes them seem more real. It also sets yourself up for expectations from friends, family, and those who you told, who will likely ask you about your progress. Don't let yourself, or them, down. Work that butt off!

BEFORE

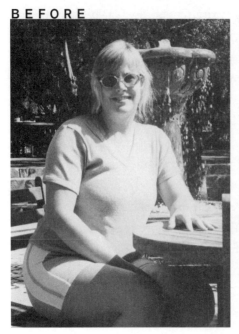

AFTER

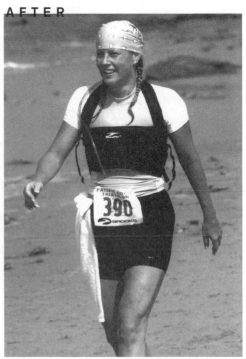

Changed My Life . . .

Loretta Petersen, 39, Los Angeles, shed 10 dress sizes with Cardio Barre.

Loretta's youngest child had just turned two, yet her last 40 baby pounds were still resiliently holding on. Desperate to slim down and strip off the fat that bulged around her bra straps, pouched around her thighs, and added an extra layer of padding on her butt, she made an appointment to have an initial consultation with a liposuction doctor. With a pile of information and the promise of sucking her thin, Loretta left the doctor and began to read through the daunting stack of facts and pre-op to-do and not-to-do lists. Despite her desire to rid the weight, all of the material scared her. Still she felt as though she had no other option. But before going under the knife, a friend introduced her to Cardio Barre, and her body, mental state, and life almost instantly improved.

Before we go into Loretta's life-altering experience with Cardio Barre, let's back up a bit. When Loretta was in college she was always the one who was asked to dance last. While her girlfriends floated along the dance floor in the arms of their beaus, Loretta dejectedly stood as a wallflower looking on. She wasn't fat, but, in her eyes, she wasn't thin enough to wear jeans. In fact, she didn't own any. Instead, she wore skirts to cover her butt. Loretta lacked self-esteem and confidence, a feeling of inadequacy that only grew worse over the years.

Okay, now fast forward to the present, actually, to two years ago. Loretta's girlfriend told her about Cardio Barre, a new exercise studio that had recently opened just a few blocks from her home. Though only in its infancy, Cardio Barre already had lines out the door of eager exercisers seeking to slim down. Being a ballet-based program, leg extensions and pliés were part of the package. The only problem was that Loretta could barely lift her leg to the barre (which is about waist high). The morning after her first class, she awoke feeling so sore that even squatting over the toilet was difficult to her utterly exhausted muscles (a sensation that sometimes recurs when she really pushes herself in class). But with some knowledge of exercise, she knew that the ache was actually a buildup of lactic acid, and that movement would help flush it out faster—as painful as it was. She returned a few days later, then maintained a schedule of taking class twice a week. Because physical change is not instantaneous with exercise, Loretta decided to give herself one year to see noticeable improvements in her body before she would go back to the liposuction doctor. Within 2 months her body was already drastically different.

Finding the motivation to keep up with her exercise program was easy. Loretta kept a picture of her pre–Cardio Barre body, reminding her of the changes that she so badly wanted to make. The image of her old self was enough to drag her tired, achy body out of bed every morning. Soon the soreness was replaced with a surge of energy, increased self-esteem, and an overall sentiment of exhilaration. The more she exercised, the more feel-good endorphins were released from her brain, and the more she wanted to exercise. Now Loretta maintains a 6-day workout week (sometimes 7-day when she feels like she really needs it). Her body now craves the endorphins, almost like an addiction, as Loretta refers to it, but it is a healthy one. She doesn't go crazy and work out aggressively all day long. Her 50-minute Cardio Barre sessions are all she needs for a good, healthy fix.

Loretta's hips have significantly shrunk. Her baby fat has gone from her waist. Her cheeks are thinning, dramatically changing her face. Her head feels better, as her self-esteem continues to be fortified. Of course, this transformation has not gone unnoticed. Loretta has been confronted with both support and criticism. Friends who have cheered her on, some of whom stood beside her on the barre, sweating right along with her, applaud her weight loss and confidence gain. But, as is a common deterrent to change, some like the "old" Loretta better, insisting that she was "more fun" when she was eating junk food and didn't have to get up early to exercise.

More important than the opinion of a few naysayers, who, to be honest, are probably just envious of Loretta's drastically improved mental and physical state, is the support of her family. A sixteen-year marriage to a wonderfully supportive husband (she is a lucky one for that) and as the mother of two kids, Loretta's weight-loss success side-effect is the ability to be a more patient mom and loving wife. As much as her husband may prefer her to stay in bed and snuggle on the weekends, instead of popping up bright and early, putting her exercise clothes on, and heading out for her 50-minute pick-me-up at Cardio Barre, he appreciates the renewed woman that she has become. An appreciation that he expressed in a beautiful letter acknowledging that women her age, after having two kids and over a decade of wedded bliss, aren't necessarily gung ho about taking care of themselves anymore. But, as he was well aware, Loretta's dedication to exercise was more than the pursuit of a perfect body, but the determination to maintain her health, so that she can physically and mentally be fully present for her family for a very long time. Every day that she exercises she is adding days to her life so that, eventually, she can add even more years to be there for her children.

Yes, being a full-time mom can be emotionally and physically exhausting. It is easy to feel like you are always giving, giving, giving, and rarely getting back in return. Loretta's exercise is a gift that she gives to herself everyday. Once her kids come home from school and her attention is again directed entirely to them, she knows that she has already done something for herself that day, which allows her to give her kids even more.

Loretta has recently adopted the name "Exercise Mom," thanks to her kids. Her son is no stranger to the gym. Even when he was an infant, Loretta toted him along to class. As she worked her butt off at the barre, he quietly sat in his baby carrier right beside her, watching in awe as his mom shed pounds of weight and even more emotional baggage. Not only did it allow Loretta the opportunity to introduce her son to a healthy lifestyle at a very, very young age, she also saved money by not having to hire a sitter. She was able to do something for herself, while still being an attentive and loving mom.

Last year, when Loretta's son was in kindergarten, he felt like sharing Mommy's healthy body practice with his voluptuous teacher, a lesson that his teacher told Mommy about. To help his teacher shed a few extra inches, Loretta's seven-year-old son suggested that his teacher got to Cardio Barre, like Mommy does!

Daddy also notices how much Loretta's body, and mind, have improved, thanks to Cardio Barre. When her husband comes home from a long day of work, and tells Loretta how pretty she looks, she has, in a sense, given herself that compliment, or, in the least, she allowed herself to receive it. And instead of being absolutely exhausted and feeling void of the ability to give much more and instead of depending on someone else to give to her, Loretta is genuinely happy, understanding, and less demanding of emotional reinforcement. Their relationship is healthier because she is more understanding and less needy. As much as compliments are always welcome, they are no longer essential to maintain Loretta's emotional self. Doing something, every day, for herself has made Loretta no longer need the extra attention from others.

Through her dedication to diet and exercise, Loretta has shed 10 dress sizes, increased muscle tone and definition, and reshaped her body . . . no liposuction needed! It may have taken a little longer than it could have had the lipo doctor gone in with his scalpel, but Loretta is empowered to know that she lost the weight herself. Her new daily routine produced changes more profound than fat loss; she gained life. She now lives life to the fullest, even in the little things. When she ventured into Gap one day and decided to try on a pair of jeans "just to see" how they looked, the sales gal insisted that her selected size was too baggy, insisting that she needed a size 6. Loretta assumed that a 6 was an impossibility. But when the sales gal returned, size 6 in hand, Loretta feverishly tried the jeans on, buttoned them up, and they fit! They weren't even the stretchy material, expanding to allow for a little extra give. Having last squeezed into a size 16, and just *because* she was now a size 6, Loretta bought the jeans—her first size-6 purchase ever! Now she owns twenty pairs of jeans, all of which remind her of how great she looks today. To maintain perspective, Loretta still has a few size 16s hanging in her closet. Sometimes she tries them on just to experience the joy of watching them fall off and to remind her that, though she may have a few flaws (in her eyes), she has come a long way baby! Loretta has learned the importance of appreciating the here and now because it doesn't get any better than today.

To challenge her physical and mental strength even more, Loretta took exercise to the ocean, and the bicycle seat, and the road, running her first triathlon. She had never swam in the ocean before, in fact, she was scared to death of it. She was in the best shape of her life and felt like, if not now, then when? To train for this ultimate test of will and strength, Loretta jogged a bit on the treadmill in addition to her regular Cardio Barre classes (and Cardio Barre tape, when she traveled). Days before the date of the race, Loretta's fear of the ocean and fear of failure began to build on her shoulders. But it wasn't necessarily about the race. Whether she decided to do it, or not, the fact was that she had ventured out of her comfort zone, challenged her mind and her body, and attempted to do something that she had never in her life imagined she would. It hadn't even crossed her mind. Yet she had already accomplished so much. And despite her fears, Loretta did gather enough courage and confidence. As exhausting and trying as the swimming, running, and biking were, Loretta completed the triathlon. It took my breath away.

I like to ask my clients to periodically take little personal tests, for themselves, so they can see where they stand. Now I am going to ask you to do this. I never ask you the number of push-ups, sit-ups, or butt raises that you do, but I do want you to know it for yourself, so that you can see how far you have come.

Loretta came up to me after one class and all she had to say was "forty." She had accomplished forty "man-style," as she calls them, push-ups. It is important to be able to give yourself a pat on the back once in a while, allowing yourself a moment to acknowledge all that you have accomplished. And if you want to go out and buy yourself a new, midriff-showing top to celebrate your success, go for it. You work hard; you deserve a reward.

12

Week Six — Mind Your Body

Do you want to be good, or great? If your answer is what I think it is, read on. . . . Let's achieve greatness together. There is no turning back. Look how far you have already come! Time is one of the most precious things in life, your health is the other. There is no time to waste. Let's take charge of our health, of our lives, and live life to the fullest. I promise that once you get physically fit, your life will change in almost every aspect.

We all want to believe that we are special in our own way and can make a difference. And we can. Each one of us brings our own uniqueness to life. This all starts with harnessing your own power and potential. Allow your light to come to life.

When you do something, especially when it concerns taking care of yourself, do it all the way, to the fullest. That is how you become the best you, you can be! Don't you want people to see the best you? Let's show them.

We never want to settle for anything in life. No settling! Why should we, when we all have the right to have it all and deserve to have it all?

It is not always easy. It is sometimes painful. But the rewards far exceed the price you pay for having all that you desire from life. In fact, you can no longer afford not to look good, feel good, and live a healthier lifestyle. This life is all that you have right now. Treasure it. Take care of it. Nurture it.

Fitness has more beneficial, long-lasting gifts to bestow than any other single thing in the world. And these gifts are priceless. The energy I wake up with and maintain throughout every day is priceless. The confidence I wake up with every morning to seize the day is priceless. The physical and mental strength I use to conquer every challenge is priceless. So are you.

So no more settling, no more limitations. Let's get to work.

MOVE YOUR BODY: WEEK SIX—5 DAYS, 50 MINUTES

The sections in this sixth week will include:
Warm-up
Pliés
Torso Twist
Cardio
Barre Thighs
Abdominals
Upper Body
Stretch

This is about the time that you should be jumping for joy, thrilled by all that you have accomplished so far, and excited about all that you will accomplish in the near future. You can never turn back now. This week we will increase your workouts by 10 minutes so that you are working out 5 days this week, for 50 minutes each session. Did you ever imagine that you would have come so far in such a short amount of time? If you have kept with the program, you are getting so much stronger, your endurance has improved tremendously, and you are feeling unstoppable. Do not compare yourself, your abilities, or performance with anyone else. This is all about you. Your journey is unique and personal to you.

See forward progress and look past all obstacles. Adopt an "I know I can" philosophy and not an "I can't" attitude. Believe you can succeed and you will.

If I have the belief that I can do it,
I shall surely acquire the capacity to do it,
even if I may not have it at the beginning.

—Mahatma Gandhi

We will add one new section this week to your routine: Abdominals. The Abdominal exercises will be added to your routine directly after the Barre Thighs exercises. Other than the extra added abs, the rest of your routine will be exactly the same as last week. If you are ready, let's do this!

–Abdominals–

Do you want a flat stomach? Who doesn't? Ninety percent of all women are dissatisfied with some aspect of their bodies. The number one complaint area is the midsection. Yup, you are not alone. The majority of women say that having a flatter and tighter midsection is at the top of their bodily wish list. People spend millions of dollars every year on abdominal exercise contraptions. You would think that everyone would be walking around with a tight, lean waistline. But, unfortunately, this is not the case. These gadgets will do little to flatten your stomach because they do little to remove the layer of fat that lies on top of your abs.

In order to trim your waistline you must understand how your abs function and how your body burns fat. Fat is excess calories stored in multiple layers on top of your muscle tissue. The muscle that the fat is stored on is made of fibers that contract to produce movement. Contrary to popular belief, fat cannot turn into muscle and muscle cannot turn into fat. You can, however, lose muscle and gain fat. In fact, losing muscle but gaining fat is, unfortunately, more common than not. So, in order to lean your waistline you must decrease the layers of fat that lie on top of it. How? Strength training, cardio, and stabilizing your blood sugar by maintaining a healthy diet.

Let's start slimmin'!

−Abdominals Section One−

The rectus abdominus is the row of washboardlike muscles in the center of your midsection. A muscularly sculpted rectus abdominus is what people are referring to when they say that someone has "six-pack" abs. They are the primary muscles used in a sit-up or crunch, pulling your chest toward your pelvis. But enough talk, it's time to work.

REGULAR CRUNCH

■ Lie on your back with your knees bent and feet flat on the ground. Placing your legs in this bent position will flatten your lumbar curve and take all the pressure off your lower back.

■ Your legs should be shoulder-width apart.

■ Place your arms in a criss-cross position across your chest with your hands loosely lying on your shoulders.

■ This is your starting position.

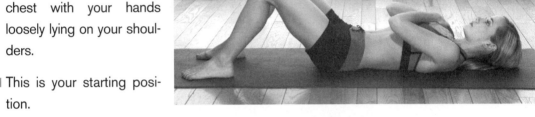

■ Contract the upper section of your abdominals, exhale, and lift your shoulders and upper torso off the ground. This is a small movement. You do not need to come to a full-seated position. In fact, your lower back should remain flat and firmly planted on the floor throughout this entire exercise.

■ Be sure to keep your neck extended, avoiding any tension or contraction. Do not fold your chin forward. This exercise is being propelled by your stomach only.

■ Once you are at the top of the sit-up, lower down to the floor without letting your shoulders completely relax down. Inhale.

■ Exhale and lift.

■ Repeat this exercise until your muscles fatigue.

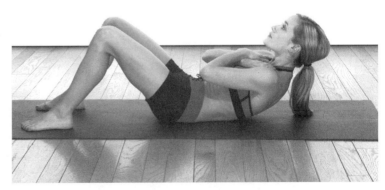

CROSS CRUNCH

- Begin in the starting position of the regular crunch. You should be lying on your back with your knees bent and feet flat on the ground. Your arms are crisscrossed across your chest with your hands on your shoulders.

- Instead of lifting your torso straight up through the center, you will be lifting side to side.

- First, lead with your right shoulder, lifting it toward your left knee. Again, do not lift your lower back off the ground. This movement is small and concentrated.

- Lower back down to your starting position, keeping your shoulders off the ground.

- Alternate sides. You will next lift your left shoulder, twisting it to your right knee. Then again your right shoulder to your left knee.

- Repeat this exercise until your muscles fatigue.

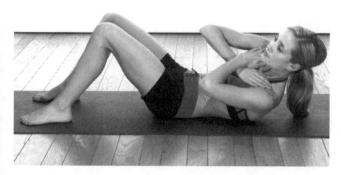 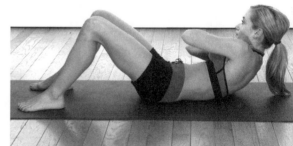

BICYCLE CRUNCH

■ Lie on your back with your knees bent, your thighs pressed up against your chest and your feet raised off the ground.

■ Place your hands behind your head, bending your elbows out to your sides. Do not grip your head or neck. This is a light touch. Any tension that you may have should be placed in your abs.

■ This is your starting position.

■ Lift your upper body off the floor by contracting your upper abdominals, pressing your lower back flat against the floor, and lifting your shoulders.

■ Twist your right shoulder to your left side as you simultaneously extend your right leg out straight in front of you without touching the ground. Your right elbow should be pointing toward your left knee as your left elbow drops back, staying in a straight line with your left torso. The lower your leg is to the ground, the harder your stomach muscles have to work, the faster you will burn the fat off your muscles and see results.

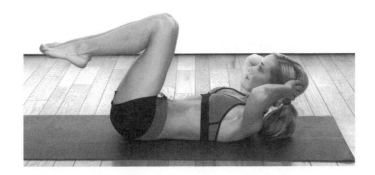

■ Lower back down to your starting position, momentarily pausing in Flat Back on the floor.

■ Pass through the center position and switch sides, twisting your left shoulder to your right side as you straighten your left leg out in front of you. Focus on lengthening one side of the waist as you contract the other. This is a slow and controlled movement, allowing you to focus on your core. I love this particular ab exercise because you are working all the muscles in the abdominal region—upper, lower, and obliques.

■ Repeat this exercise until your muscles fatigue. As you gain strength, you will be able to increase your reps. Of course, the more the better, but do not jeopardize the integrity of the movement just to add a few extra reps. Doing the exercise wrong will only increase your risk of injury. It is less about how many reps you do, and more about how many you do correctly. Working full range of motion at a high intensity will enable you to do fewer reps with faster results!

−Abdominals Section Two−

Reverse crunches are a great exercise for the lower rectus abdominus. Usually the lower abdominals are less developed than the upper abs. They are often the pouch that bulges out below your belly button. It is time to tame that excess fat!

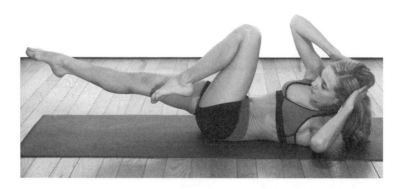

REVERSE CRUNCH

■ Lie on your back with your arms straight along your sides, palms down.

■ Raise your feet off the floor and bend your knees to a 90-degree angle from your torso. Your thighs should be perpendicular to the floor, your calves parallel to the floor, and your feet raised in the air.

■ Squeeze your legs together.

■ This is your starting position.

■ Lift your hips off the floor by contracting your lower abs and pulling your knees up and into your chest. Your hips will rise a couple of inches off the floor.

■ Maintaining the contraction in your abs, slowly lower your legs and hips to your starting position.

■ Your head and neck should remain flat and relaxed against the floor.

■ Repeat this exercise until your muscles are fatigued.

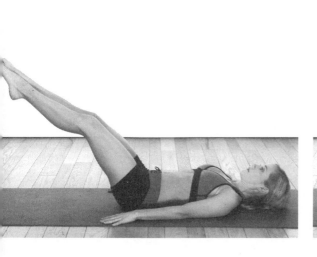
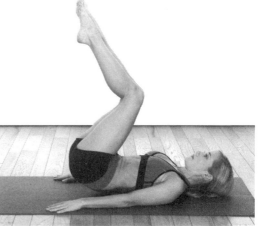

SIDE CRUNCHES

■ Your obliques are the muscles that help you bend side to side and rotate your torso. When you refer to your "love handles," you are talking about the fat deposits in the oblique area. Let's get rid of them!

■ Lie on you back with your legs together, knees bent, and feet on the floor.

■ Allow your legs to fall over to your left side so the left leg is resting on the floor and the right knee is directly above the left. Your torso should be slightly twisted but both shoulders should be firmly planted on the floor.

■ Place your hands behind your head with a light touch.

■ This is your starting position.

■ Contract your abs and raise your head and shoulders off the floor. Do not raise your lower back off the floor.

■ Hold in that position for 2 seconds.

■ Lower down to the starting position.

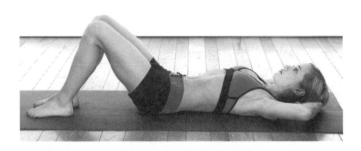

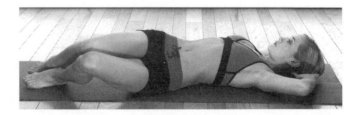

■ Hold in that position for 2 seconds.

■ Repeat the side crunches on your left side until your muscles fatigue.

■ Switch sides, twisting your knees to your right side.

■ Contract your abs and raise your head and shoulders off the floor. Do not raise your lower back off the floor.

■ Hold in the starting position for 2 seconds.

■ Lower down to the starting position.

■ Hold in the starting position for 2 seconds.

■ Repeat the side crunches on your right side until your muscles fatigue.

BEFORE   **AFTER**

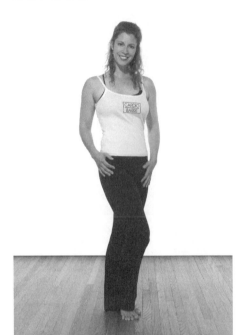 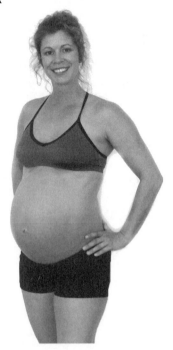

Changed My Life . . .

Helena Talman, 32, a Radio City Rockette, did Cardio Barre throughout her pregnancy.

Helena did Cardio Barre up to the ninth month of her pregnancy. A lot of women do. Working out during pregnancy is not only good for the body, but it is amazing for your mind. Of course, if you have never worked out a day in your life, jumping into an intense 5-day a-week program is probably not recommended; but for someone like Helena, it was what her body needed.

Helena is a very active person. She always has been. In fact, she turned physical activity into her career. Each winter she heads to New York, puts on a little red dress with white cuffs, and kicks her legs really high performing as a Radio City Rockette for their Christmas show. Obviously, in order to be a Rockette, your body must be stunning and strong. To stay in shape during her off months, Helena depended on both cardio and strength training. She is also a Pilates instructor and massage therapist in Los Angeles, originally from Sweden. Getting outdoors and breathing in some fresh air is important to her, so when not in a gym, Helena hikes. Clearly, she did not seek out Cardio Barre to shed a whole lot of pounds. Helena actually came to Cardio Barre out of boredom. Okay, I admit, at first she was skeptical. Her husband bought her a gift certificate to take a class. Having taken just about every new class in the city, and testing every fitness trend—from Tae Bo to urban trekking and Spinning—she definitely had her doubts that this dance-based class would have the ability to peak and keep her interest.

When so many classes are purported to be the best, and you bought into each "best" promise, only to be disappointed by its shortcomings, your trust in "best" begins to wane. Thankfully, Helena's husband is an old friend of mine, and he was able to convince her to finally just check out the class. If she hated it, at least she gave it a shot. Luckily, she loved it! Despite the fact that she is a dancer, Helena still felt challenged. Her daily exercise regimen used to consist of both a strength and cardio workout, but now she was getting a two-for-one deal, cutting her workout time and increasing the benefits. And after only a few classes, she was surprised to see changes in her body. He lean dancers' legs were lengthened even more. She loved to watch her butt steadily rise, her core strength continue to strengthen, and her stamina increase. Even other Rockettes commented on her ability to keep on kicking during show rehearsals and shows without tiring. Her team captain noticed her arms—they were long and lean, but her muscles were cut and incredibly strong. Kicking over and over again as a Rockette is exhausting, but Cardio Barre was able to increase Helena's kick-ability! Soon, other LA-based Rockettes joined Helena in their off seasons to keep their bodies in optimum shape throughout the year—even when not dancing for 10 hours a day. Sometimes Helena's husband would join too, which was always a boost for her. At the end of class he was soaked in sweat and the next morning only ibuprofen could relieve his sore muscles.

In many ways, Helena found that Cardio Barre was similar to Pilates in that it works to strengthen the core. Her über-body understanding and alignment awareness, thanks to both her Pilates and massage-therapy training, gives

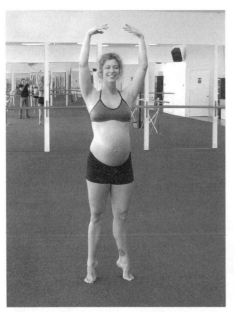 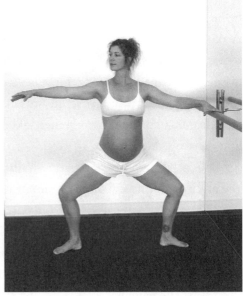

Helena a, shall we say, leg up when it comes to knowing if certain movements are good or jarring for the body, muscles, and bones. When taking classes that focus on kicking and punching, for example, Helena could feel that she was jeopardizing the health of her body, potentially setting herself up for injury. In fact, many of her clients come to her for massage when in major pain from throwing their bodies out in one of those other classes. Their bodies are destroyed, they can barely move, and they don't know why. With any exercise program, you have to keep in mind that, while you may be strong, you are not invincible. Don't be hardheaded when it comes to the health of your bodies. If you feel like a movement is off, it probably is. Don't push it. When you do such impacting exercises, it is easy to throw out a joint. When you are constantly crunching and contracting your muscles, without giving them enough of a stretch or expansion, you are left with short, stubby, bulky muscles—definitely not what a Rockette can dance with, especially if she can't even walk thanks to an exercise-induced injury! Helena's body and its ability to move fluidly is her career; she has to be especially careful not to mistreat it. That's why she does Cardio Barre.

What is great for me personally to see is the music moving through my students. In class, you can tell that Helena is in her element. The music starts blaring and her toes start pointing, her fingers shape into that of a dancer, and when those legs start kicking—watch out! Even though she is a dancer by trade, the other non-dancers in class—the housewives, attorneys, actresses, and school teachers—are learning to be just as graceful, strong, lean, and flexible. The movements are structured in such a way that, even if you don't know what a Plié is, you will by the end of the first class. Watching so many women, of all ages and ability, taking care of themselves and putting energy into the upkeep of their bodies and minds, is so inspiring.

More than the physical benefits of Cardio Barre, Helena, like most of my students, continues to come back to class because of what it does for her emotionally. I literally hear this everyday: "I need Cardio Barre for my sanity." To be honest, I have had more than a couple of husbands actually thank me for Cardio Barre. Yeah, they love that their wives have firm behinds and slim waistlines because of the class, but it is often the mental aspect that the men most appreciate. Helena's husband knows the importance of those 50 minutes a day that she dedicates to herself in class. In fact, if she is in a bad mood, her husband asks her to go relax at Cardio Barre. Not that a class is necessarily relaxing in the sense that we just sit around and give each other back massages; it is relaxing in that you momentarily escape from the craziness of life, get a good sweat, pump up your self-esteem, and walk out feeling like a strong, beautiful woman.

You don't have to be in Los Angeles in one of my classes in order to feel the benefits of Cardio Barre. When traveling to Sweden to visit her mom, Helena makes sure to bring the Cardio Barre tape in her carry-on. She got her mom hooked too. About twice a week, they move the couches, set up two chairs (as stand-ins for a barre), drop a towel on the ground, pop the tape into the VCR, and start sweating. At first, her mom didn't have the endurance to do the class in its entirety, though who would expect her to when attempting to tackle a new form of movement? She would sit out during the really hard stuff, sometimes take a break halfway; but after a couple of classes, she was sweating through the entire class! Of course, she had it harder than students in class, because using a chair as opposed to a barre makes it tough to cheat. With something really sturdy, like a barre or kitchen counter, you can put too much weight on it, relinquishing some stability to the barre instead of creating it within your body, which makes the class easier—but that is cheating. With a chair, you can only put so much pressure on it, and that "so much" is very little. Instead of holding on to it for support, you are forced to hold your stomach for support, strengthening your core even more. That is when you really feel it in your abs and butt! Helena's mom now has her own tape, so she doesn't have to depend on her daughter's visits to get her workout in.

When Helena found out she was pregnant, she figured that, since she had seen other pregnant women in class, if they could do it, so could she. But, just to be sure, she checked with her doctor first. Because she was a regular exerciser, even before the pregnancy, there was no reason to stop, except with a little modification here and there. For the first few months Helena came to class wearing a heart monitor to ensure that her heart rate didn't spike too high. Sometimes her heart would really speed up, and she would just take herself down a bit until she felt comfortable, but she wouldn't stop moving. Dizzy spells sometimes struck Helena, especially during the first few months. So she upped her water intake and opted to ease off on the intensity a little. As she progressed in her pregnancy, and her belly got bigger, she had to cut out the sit-ups and drop down from taking class twice a week to once a week. When she began her ninth month, Helena stopped taking class. A few weeks later she went into an easy labor, by most standards, and popped out that baby in just 5½ hours! Her doctors had told her that she would enjoy a fast and easy labor, thanks to being in such great shape, but couldn't believe just how fast and easy it was!

Of course, everyone is different and all pregnancies are unique. While Helena was able to continue taking class for most of her pregnancy, and her level of fitness and core strength assisted in a quick and relatively easy birth, she has dancer friends who were sick as dogs throughout the entirety of their pregnancies, unable to leave their house much, let alone exercise. But for Helena, exercise made her feel good, and in the end, that is the most important thing. Don't do something because someone else says you should do it, or because "everyone else is doing it," do things that you want to do because they make you feel good. Though, I have never run into anyone who flat out says that exercise makes them feel bad. Sure, maybe during the actual act of exercising, someone will look up at me and tell me that they are "never taking my class again" because they are struggling though a difficult section of the class. But, after the class, they always have a smile on their face as they exclaim "see you tomorrow" or "see you next week!"

It has been a month since Helena gave birth, and she is already getting back into class to reclaim her pre-pregnancy shape.

13

Week Seven — Mind Your Body

Two more weeks and you have put yourself on the road to your perfect body! Can you believe this? What an accomplishment already! How are you feeling? What changes have occurred in your life? Have your friends and family noticed? How can they not? Not only is your body slimming and toning, but your mind is changing, your attitude and outlook are evolving, and you are developing into the person that you have always wanted to be. Your attitude, enthusiasm, and self-confidence are all critical to success because a winning attitude energizes your mission, transforming raw potential into sheer power. On the other hand, a negative, self-defeating attitude destroys all hope of success—personally and professionally. If you want a better career, better relationships, a better life, you have to embrace this attitude adjustment that you are experiencing. You have begun on your path to success, in fact, you have already experienced much success along this path, but just because this book is about to end does not mean that it is time for your exploration of your potential has to end. This is just the beginning of the brand-new you.

This very well may not be the first time that you have tried to make change, but it is likely the first time that the change that you are making has reached your depths. This kind of change sticks with you . . . if you continue to work on it. It is not fleeting; it won't turn around and bite you in the butt. If you stick with everything that you have learned, maintaining your new food and fitness attitude and allowing it to continue to be a regular part of your life, a lifestyle really, you will only find more and more success. Sometimes it just takes a little extra push, an oomph of energy from an outside source that propels you to finally take action and explore your potential. Don't stop exploring. Never settle for "good enough." Because, you know what? "Good enough" isn't. Comfort shouldn't be comfortable. Mediocrity should not be your goal. Milk this life of yours for all it is. Be the absolute best that you can be. Push your limits. Break through boundaries. And by all means, DON'T SETTLE!

We know where your head is. Where is your body? I know that you have worked your body beyond your preconceived limitations. Throughout the past 6 weeks, your muscles may have felt like they were ripping. You may have cried out in frustration and in fear of self-defeat. You probably stumbled upon your breaking point. But you surpassed it. You may have popped multiple Tylenol just to get to sleep at night, only to wake to screaming muscles in the morning. You have undoubtedly suffered from pain, frustration, and multiple loads of sweat soaked laundry. How are you feeling now? Are you exuding confidence from each and every one of your pores? You should be. You have worked your butt off, literally—feel proud. I am proud of you. Are you allowing yourself to acknowledge how far you have come? Are you giving yourself that well-deserved pat on the back, that sexy new outfit, or a night on the town to celebrate? Okay, don't go too crazy, we still have 2 weeks to go. But give yourself a little slack, flash that winning smile, and flaunt your new body and attitude. Success is oh-so-sweet. Drink it in!

Far better is it to dare mighty things, to win glorious triumphs, even though checkered by failure . . . than to rank with those poor spirits who neither enjoy much nor suffer much, because they live in a gray twilight that knows not victory nor defeat.

—THEODORE ROOSEVELT

MOVE YOUR BODY: WEEK SEVEN—6 DAYS, 50 MINUTES

The sections in this second week will include:
Warm-up
Pliés
Torso Twist
Cardio
Barre Thighs
Abdominals
Upper Body
Stretch

It is time to take your workout to another level. We are about to add an extra exercise day to your week. Yes, you will be working out 6 days a week! This is amazing! Would you ever have imagined that exercise would actually be a part of your life—a lifestyle? The answer to that question is "yes." You did imagine it or else you would not be doing it right now. It is all about setting your sights high, but taking baby steps to get there. You have a tremendous amount of courage and determination, or else you would not have aspired to this level of greatness and, without aspiring, you would never have gotten here. Keep your focus. Talk to others who have accomplished through hardships yet pulled through to attain success. Learn from them and let them motivate you. Don't dwell on the complainers who constantly seem to fail. Learn from the "doers," because you have proven yourself to be a doer too! You will repeat the same routine as in Week Five, but you will add one more day to your workout.

BEFORE

AFTER

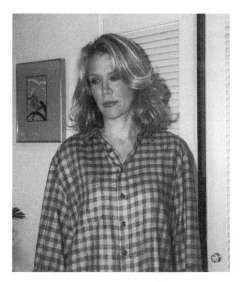

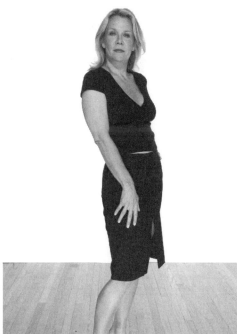

Changed My Life . . .

Kaden Foster, 53, eased arthritis, left an unhealthy relationship, and made her way back into the working world through the strength she found in Cardio Barre.

A few years ago, Kaden's husband died of brain cancer. She fell into a deep depression. Feeling alone and desperate for someone to hold her, she started a fun little fling to ease her loneliness. It was supposed to be a brief interlude, but it dragged on for years. To make matters worse, she was diagnosed with arthritis in her hip, an inherited ailment, minimizing her range of motion and further crippling her self-esteem. Weight had never been a serious problem for Kaden, but once in a while it would have a tendency to creep up. This was one of those "once in a while" occasions. Since she had always had a lot of animals, and walking dogs was a regular occurrence, she had never developed a traditional exercise regimen. In order to control her weight and ease her stress, it was time to find one.

Without missing a beat, Kaden bought a membership to a gym, hired a personal trainer, and prepared to finally emerge from this extended bout of depression that had subtly filled the past several years of her life. While many of the other gym-goers sauntered along the rows of exercise equipment, perfectly clad in designer fitness wear, and with the air and appearance most often seen at red carpet arrivals to Hollywood events, Kaden took her workout seriously. Who had bigger muscles and whose workout gear was more in style was of no interest to her. It wasn't about seeing and being seen, it was about finding her muscles and increasing her endurance. Unfortunately, her personal trainers (all struggling actors) were more interested in acting like trainers (and making sure everyone was watching) than actually training. After going through a few "trainers," Kaden felt more dread in entering the social scene that the gym was clearly mistaken for than excitement in unveiling her healthier, stronger, happier self. She faced the fact that her gym experience lacked the sense of camaraderie that she needed to motivate and maintain a routine . . . so she quit.

A few months later, a friend convinced Kaden to try out a new exercise craze called Cardio Barre. Considering that the studio was 40 minutes away (at least an hour in traffic) it took a little convincing to get this non-dancer to go out of her way to endure a ballet-based exercise class. Finally, she gave in and decided to try it out. She showed up in old comfy sweatpants, and was thrilled to find out that she perfectly fit in with the rest of the class. Cardio Barre is anything but pretentious. Everyone is there to work out . . . period. Of course, there is a social element to it, as there is with any group setting. But it isn't about "who looks better," instead it is about friendships and support. Some students are professional dancers, and some have never felt an ounce of grace in their entire lives. And that is okay. Everyone starts somewhere.

Kaden's first class was, and I am being nice, a bit of a struggle for her. Okay, in her words, "It was horrible!" She could not keep up. She held on to the barre for her life and she could barely lift her arthritic leg. But she absolutely loved it, and she wanted more! Despite her difficulty and apparent lack of balance, after that one hour, Kaden could feel a bit of a dancer emerging from her depths. She felt elegant and sexy and feminine. Sweat poured from her pores and, by the end of class, her face was beet red and she had the purest smile of sheer joy and accomplishment beaming from cheek to cheek.

Though Kaden had always considered herself to be a klutz, she had finally found a program that excited her, offered a sense of camaraderie, challenged her body and mind, and was an outlet for stress release. With the mantra The Only Time You Fail Is When You Quit, Kaden, who was definitely not a quitter, kept it up, knowing that she could only get better each time. A few days later, she was back in class.

Because many of the movements in class are based on ballet movements, all of which were unfamiliar to Kaden's body, she depended on the barre to maintain her balance and keep her from falling. But with each class, as her core slowly but surely gained strength, she was able to depend on herself for balance. She found that she could lift her leg slightly higher and she began to feel increasingly flexible. After a few months, she was able to focus on certain muscle groups, consciously deciding if she wanted to put the stretch in her core or her thighs, or if she preferred to feel her muscles burn in her hamstrings or butt. Once you are in touch with your body, it is easy to become acutely aware of what muscles are working at what time. Put your mind on your muscle and your muscle will respond.

For Kaden, it was, at first, a challenge to really quiet her mind enough to hear her body. But that one hour of time that she dedicated to herself, to listening to what her muscles were saying and learning to have the ability to tell a certain body part to move, imagining an increase of blood flow to that area, and having her blood respond by going to that area, is when she really saw change. Once Kaden learned to quiet her mind and listen to her body, she would sometimes look up in the middle of an exercise and see her reflection in the mirror and actually be surprised that she was looking at herself—that she looked so good, so graceful, and so defined. Sometimes the change is that quick, and it actually surprises you.

In each class, Kaden pushed herself just a little bit further. But there is one position in particular that continued to be a challenge to her—plank. Plank is the top of a push-up. You hold your body flat, parallel to the ground. Your arms remain straight, perpendicular to the ground. Your entire body weight is supported only by your hands and toes. It may sound easy, but after holding it for a few seconds, your stomach muscles quickly tire as your arms begin to shake from exhaustion. In this one position, you are working your entire body. Kaden came to view plank as a measure of her strength, both physical and mental. When she was in a difficult situation outside of class, she would think to herself, "If I can hold plank, I can do anything!" Because of her arthritis, whenever in plank, a tear filled her left eye, shooting straight from her left hip. But Cardio Barre has actually significantly helped her arthritis. In fact, when she skips class, her hip acts up. She is a testament of the fact that exercise helps arthritis. It is extremely therapeutic and strengthening.

As Kaden's body evolved, so did her mind. She began to view herself as a strong, beautiful woman. She realized that, for so long, she had existed under a dark veil of mourning, despite the fact that she had physically moved on and maintained her relationship with her "fling." Within the unhealthy comfort of this relationship, Kaden had never allowed herself to completely heal and be happy. Once her body began to strengthen, her self-esteem began to rise, and she started listening to the things that I said over and over in class—"You deserve all of life's happiness. Never settle for good enough when you can have the best!"

Instead of sitting around, allowing her life to pass her by, Kaden decided to update her self-image. She realized that she had become introverted and no longer accomplished much . . . because she didn't feel like she could and she had found comfort in mediocrity. But there is a time when your comfort zone is not good enough and you have to move on. Kaden had come to that time. She realized that this man who had become her long-lasting "little fling," didn't deserve her. Finally, after years of having settled in the "comfort" of this man's arms, she realized that she didn't like the way he was treating her. She thought about plank, then told him that she deserved more and that she had to leave. And she did. Cardio Barre helped Kaden liberate herself from anger, fear, and self-doubt. The relationship had become a crutch, and she finally learned how to walk on her own.

Once she had the strength to shed her unhealthy relationship, she also found the strength to embrace even more change. After ten years of not working, Kaden was struggling through plank when she came to realize that she needed to be more productive in life. The cure to ignorance is education. So, the next day, she went back to school to reinstill her skills and rejoin the workforce in the field of law. When it was time to interview for jobs, Kaden's old mind-set kicked in—"I am not good enough. They can find someone better than me. . . ." But then, she thought of plank and decided, "No, I am the best. They need me. If I don't know something, I will learn it!"

Moving out of your comfort zone can be scary, be it in business, relationships, or life. Kaden faced her fear of change head-on, and now her smile almost never falls off her face (except when she is really struggling through plank). Finding the strength within her body inspired her to push herself in all aspects of her life as she sought to achieve greatness! She swears that much of it is thanks to plank. Plank pulled her through her difficult breakup, it helped her navigate through struggles at work, and it continues to remind her of her physical and mental strength. Kaden sometimes refers to class as therapy—though it is much less expensive than therapy. And her drug of choice has become her endorphins.

All of that excess baggage that Kaden used to haul around is discarded. She doesn't need it anymore. Now, she makes room for new relationships and the better life that she creates for herself everyday. Feeling much lighter in spirit, her body is getting comfortable in its skin, shedding excess weight that is, like the baggage, no longer needed to pad her. She finally has a defined waistline and toned arms and legs. Her dress size has dropped from a size 8 to 4. With a better body and increased self-esteem, Kaden's stance has changed. She imagines that a thin string is attached to the top of her head and it is constantly pulling her up, allowing her posture to be perfect! Instead of hunching over, she now holds her shoulders back, lifts her chest, and stands as tall as her newly petite frame will allow.

At 53 years old, Kaden is often told that she looks better than she did in her 20s and 30s. But more than looking better, she feels sexier than she ever has. In fact, she exudes sexiness. Her smile is infectious and her friends love this new Kaden that has finally crawled out from the darkness of her husband's death.

She swears that Cardio Barre makes her look like she had a facelift. By the end of each class, her face is flushed, her eyes are sparkling, she is completely drenched in sweat, and her glistening skin appears to be firmer and lifted. Because your blood is pumping and so many toxins are released from your body within your sweat, your skin improves—as though you had a facial.

Cutting out alcohol and minimizing her sugar consumption has undoubtedly also contributed to Kaden's improved skin tone. Changing her diet actually comes naturally. Because Kaden wants to make every workout count as much as it possibly can, she has minimized anything that hinders her body from performing at its optimum level. Drinking alcohol, eating an excess of sugar, or a heavy meal substantially decreases Kaden's energy, as though she poured sugar in her gas tank. Of course, she can't help but splurge on a few peanut M&Ms now and then. It's all about balance. Even cheating here and there can be healthy. All in all, Kaden views Cardio Barre as her insurance plan, but this plan prevents illness instead of merely easing you through it.

14

Week Eight—Mind Your Body

Are you jumping for joy right about now? I hope I am not the only one jumping up and down. You have 1 week left. One! This is a serious accomplishment. The magnitude of this is huge! You have proven to yourself that you can succeed at anything if you put your mind to it. If that doesn't feel good, I don't know what does. But don't give up now. First of all, you have to finish this final week, and second, you have to keep it up. Don't slack off and don't celebrate by gorging yourself. You have successfully broken unhealthy patterns and created new healthy ones. You have freed yourself from unhealthy emotional attachments and self-sabotaging habits. You broke yourself down in order to put yourself back together the way you want to be seen, the way you want to feel. And look at you now. You have achieved your goal.

Don't go back. Never go back. Look forward and move forward. You have to keep up. Continue to push yourself. Change your routine to keep it interesting. If you slack off and your old body comes back, these past two hard-working months were for nothing. You wasted your time, you wasted my time. Don't waste time—work out!

Fit Tip

Millions of people suffer from back problems. Strengthening your core and back muscles reduces or eliminates most of them.

Look in the mirror. No, don't just glance, and definitely don't pick yourself apart, searching for flaws. Stand in front of the mirror and appreciate your beautiful body for all that it is. Love it for taking this journey with you. Appreciate it for succeeding, even when it wanted to give up. Wear your sexy curves like the diva that you are. You lighten up a room when you enter it. Heads turn as you walk down the street. But you don't care anymore because you honestly don't even notice. You know how hot you are, you don't need others to reaffirm that fact anymore. You feel balanced and at ease. Your body and your attitude have come a long way baby! You are like a new woman! You no longer sleepwalk through your life. That sexy, strong, self-confident woman that lay dormant within you has awoken. Watch out world!

MOVE YOUR BODY: WEEK EIGHT–6 DAYS, 60 MINUTES

The sections in this second week will include:
Warm-up
Pliés
Torso Twist
Cardio
Barre Thighs
Abdominals
Upper Body
Floor Work
Stretch

Visualize your goal because it's right in front of you! See the finish line and don't stop until you have crossed it. This is your last and final week with me, and we have upped the stakes. You will be working out 6 days this week for 60 minutes each day! This is hot! You are hot! Constantly remind yourself of your dreams and goals, and never give up.

The last and final section added will be Floor Work. These Floor Work exercises will come directly after the Upper Body.

−Floor Work−

To protect your body from any unnecessary discomfort, do Floor Work on a carpet or on an exercise mat.

The lower back is one of the most ignored muscle groups when it comes to working out. Pelvis tilts will help strengthen your lower back and narrow your waist.

PELVIS TILTS

■ Lie on your back with your knees bent and your feet flat on the floor.

■ This is your starting position.

■ Exhale as you contract your stomach muscles and lift your lower back and butt up off the floor, pressing your hips up to the ceiling. Your butt should lift approximately 6 inches off the floor. Be sure to keep your shoulders and upper back on the floor. You are essentially making a bridge.

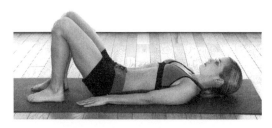

■ Once you have reached the top of the tilt, slowly lower your hips back down until your butt is approximately 1 inch from the floor. This is a controlled movement that will help strengthen your lower back and firm your butt.

■ Repeat the pelvis tilt until your muscles fatigue.

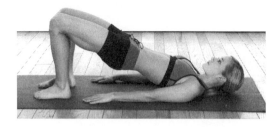

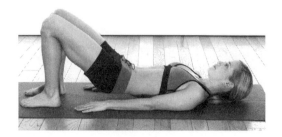

SIDE LEG LIFTS

■ Lie straight on your back.

■ Roll onto your left side, keeping your legs straight together and your feet flexed. Your left leg should be on the floor and your right leg should be on top of your left.

■ Prop your head up with your left hand as if you were watching TV.

■ Place the palm of your right hand firmly on the floor to support you.

■ This is your starting position.

■ Lift your right leg upward, creating a V shape between your right and left leg.

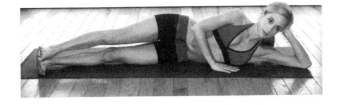

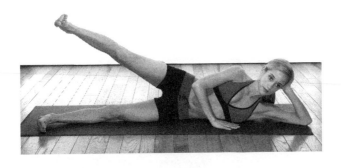

■ Lower your right leg back down until you have a 1-inch space between your legs, but do not let your right leg touch your left. Extend your legs straight the entire time in order to stretch and tone simultaneously. Focus on your outer thigh lifting and stretch through to your heel. These are excellent exercises for the thighs, hips, and butt. The secret is keeping your working leg as straight as possible so you will lengthen and strengthen the muscle at the same time. It takes a little more effort, but the payoff is worth it.

■ Do 32 reps.

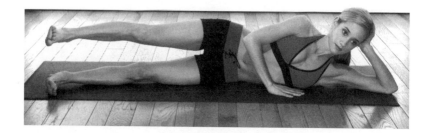

QUARTER LEG LIFTS

■ Maintain your starting position, but rotate your body a quarter turn toward the floor so that you are almost on your stomach.

■ Allow your left leg to extend slightly in front of your right so that your legs are no longer on top of each other. Point your right foot to the wall behind you.

■ Your left pelvic bone should be pressing into the floor.

■ This is your starting position.

■ Lift your right leg straight up into the air.

■ Lower your leg back down, but do not let it rest on your left leg. Maintain your body alignment by keeping your right leg directly behind your head. Do not arch your back. You are working the area around the thighs, targeting the different muscles groups in the hip, thigh, and butt areas. Remember to keep your working leg (the top leg) straight.

■ Repeat 32 times.

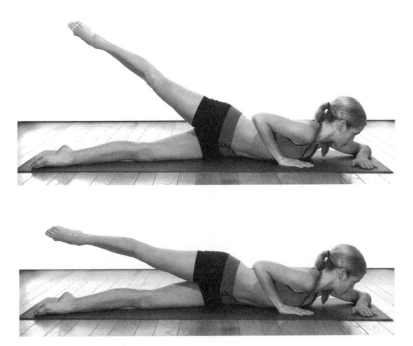

STOMACH LEG LIFTS

- Repeat the same starting position as the Quarter Leg Lifts, but rotate your body another quarter turn so that you are lying on your stomach.

- Slightly cross your legs so that your left supporting leg is in front of your right working leg.

- Lift your right leg straight up.

- Lower your right leg back down, but do not let it rest on your left. Be sure that you don't bounce your right leg on your left thigh. This is a controlled movement. The Stomach Leg Lifts target the lower butt, also known as the glutes. Lift with a consistent and controlled movement. Stomach Leg Lifts help lift the sag in your butt. It is the perfect pantyline pick-me-up!

- Lift for 32 reps.

- Hold the final rep, with your right leg raised in the air, for 8 seconds.

- Release your leg and roll onto your back.

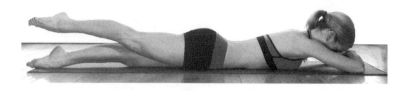

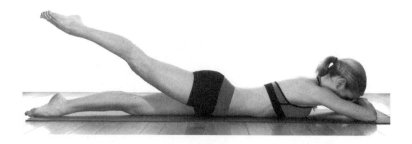

–Other Side–

PELVIS TILTS

■ Repeat the Pelvis Tilts. Lie on your back with your knees bent and your feet flat on the floor. Contract your stomach muscles and lift your lower back and butt up off the floor, pressing your hips up to the ceiling. Then lower down.

■ Repeat for 32 reps.

SIDE LEG LIFTS

■ Roll onto your right side and repeat the leg lifts using your right leg as the supporting leg and left leg as the working leg.

■ You will be on your right side, keeping your legs straight together and your feet flexed. Your right leg should be on the floor and your left leg should be on top of your right.

■ Prop your head up with your right hand as if you were watching TV.

■ Place the palm your left hand firmly on the floor to support you.

■ This is your starting position.

■ Lift your left leg upward, creating a V shape between your left and right leg.

■ Lower your left leg back down until you have a 1-inch space between your legs, but do not let your left leg touch your right. Extend your legs straight the entire time in order to stretch and tone simultaneously.

■ Do 32 reps.

QUARTER LEG LIFTS

■ Maintain your starting position, but rotate your body a quarter turn toward the floor so that you are almost on your stomach.

■ Allow your right leg to extend slightly in front of your left so that your legs are no longer on top of each other. Point your left foot to the wall behind you.

■ Your right pelvic bone should be pressing into the floor.

■ This is your starting position.

■ Lift your left leg straight up into the air.

■ Lower your leg back down, but do not let it rest on your right leg. Remember to keep your working leg (the top leg) straight.

■ Repeat 32 times.

STOMACH LEG LIFTS

■ Repeat the same starting position as the Quarter Leg Lifts, but rotate your body another quarter turn so that you are lying on your stomach.

■ Slightly cross your legs so that your right supporting leg is in front of your left working leg.

■ Lift your left leg straight up.

■ Lower your left leg back down but do not let it rest on your right. Be sure that you don't bounce your left leg on your right thigh.

■ Lift for 32 reps.

■ Hold the final rep, with your right leg raised in the air, for 8 seconds.

■ Release your leg and roll onto your back.

PELVIS TILTS

■ Repeat the Pelvis Tilts. Lie on your back with your knees bent and your feet flat on the floor. Contract your stomach muscles and lift your lower back and butt up off the floor, pressing your hips up to the ceiling. Then lower down.

■ Repeat for 32 reps.

When transitioning into each leg lift section do not stop the movement; these are done with a *continual* fat-burning motion that keeps constant stress on the muscles.

You have just worked all the way around the thighs, now let's work inner thighs. These exercises are designed to lengthen and lean out your hips and thighs. They will not bulk you up, just make you leaner and sexier! They work . . . but you have to work too.

INNER THIGHS

■ Lie on your right side with your right leg stretched straight out and your left knee bent.

■ Place your left foot on the floor just behind your right leg, pulled up as close to your butt as is comfortable.

■ Your right inner thigh should be facing upward.

■ Lift the right leg up about 1 foot off the ground.

■ Lower down. Do not let the right leg touch the floor as you are lowering it down.

■ Repeat for 32 reps.

■ Without stopping, cross your left leg over to the front of your right leg, pulling the left foot close to the front of your thigh.

■ Do 32 leg lifts.

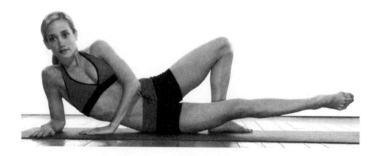

−Other Side−

INNER THIGHS

■ Lie on your left side with your left leg stretched straight out and your right knee bent.

■ Place your right foot on the floor just behind your left leg, pulled up as close to your butt as is comfortable.

■ Your left inner thigh should be facing upward.

■ Lift the left leg up about 1 foot off the ground.

> # Fit Tip
>
> For best results do not quit when you begin to fatigue. Use your mental strength to push yourself just a little further, really breaking the muscle down. REMEMBER: In order to change the muscle, you must work beyond what your body is used to. The more you work out, the further you will have to go and the more reps you may have to do. There is never an ending point in exercise . . . you can always do more and you can always push harder and go further.

■ Lower down. Do not let the left leg touch the floor as you are lowering it down.

■ Repeat for 32 reps.

■ Without stopping, cross your right leg over to the front of your left leg, pulling the right foot close to the front of your thigh.

■ Do 32 leg lifts.

Inner thigh work will help tighten and lean the flabby section on the inside of your thighs. It will also lengthen and strengthen the muscle while burning the layer of fat that sits on top. Always work both sides with the same amount of reps and the same intensity level.

During any and all sections you may increase or decrease the reps to suit your own needs, creating an easier or more challenging workout. As you get stronger you will want to add more reps or go for a longer period of time.

Remember, what you put into it is what you will get out of it. Working lazy gets you a lazy body. Working out hard gets you a hard body. The choice is yours.

This is it! You've done it! You have completed the Cardio Barre program. You have pushed yourself, you have sweat, and you have cried. Your muscles have throbbed in pain as you pressed and pulled your way out of the ruts in your life and you have raised your barre! Congratulations! I feel like I should hug you, but I can't since we are communicating through a book. So right now, I want you to wrap your arms around yourself and give yourself one big congratulatory hug! You should be proud. I am.

But just because the book is done and your 8 weeks are over doesn't mean that it is time to go back to your old ways. The only way that you can continue enjoying the changes that you have earned and worked so hard for, is by continuing to work hard for them. No, you don't need to work quite as hard. You can skip a few workouts sometimes. But you likely won't want to. I'll bet that your body feels better when it is working out, that you will actually miss the workout if you miss a workout. In terms of food choices, try to stick with what you have been doing. Again, a splurge every once in a while is okay. But, like with the exercise, I'd be willing to bet that your body feels better when you are eating well. By now, you should be in touch with yourself enough to know what your body wants and doesn't want, you should be able to understand the signals that it sends you when it is happy or not. The one thing I ask you to do is to continue listening to your body. It is the most important guide to your health. Stay healthy, lean, and happy. If you need me again, I am always here.

BEFORE

AFTER

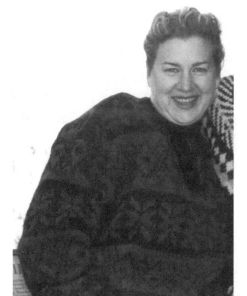

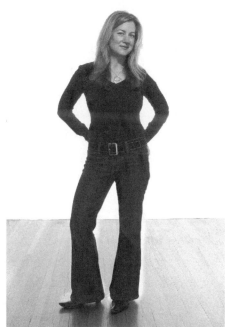

Changed My Life . . .

Francine Martin Hill, 45, raised her barre and changed her life.

Many women say that as soon as you turn 30, things change . . . particularly your body. After years of minimal maintenance to keep your naturally slim-and-trim limbs bikini ready, a new decade dawns and as the sun rises on your thirtieth birthday, so does your weight! It is as inevitable as a college girl's "freshman 15" nightmare. Francine was struck by the 30-30. But, as many 30-year-olds experience, her weight gain was not purely "right of passage" pounds; life suddenly leaped into the fast lane, creating new responsibilities, inducing unforeseen stresses, and, in turn, the pounds began to pile on.

Francine was at the height of her career and in search of a source of comfort during this time of constant transition. Aware that her nicotine habit was unhealthy, she stopped smoking, but swapped the cigarettes for another addictive substance—food. Food became her "friend," and excessive emotional eating began to reshape her body. She equates food to shoes—"food always fits," whether in a moment of weakness or strength, depression or celebration, somehow food always seemed to fit right in. Francine's once itty-bitty body ballooned from a size 5 to a size 12, yet she was in complete denial. Having been athletic and fit all her life, Francine dove into a hard-core aerobic regimen. After a few months, the weight began to come off, but her body refused to return to the svelte physique that it once was. Frustrated and exhausted, she stopped working out and watched as her weight eclipsed her pre-exercise size. Without enough hours in the day to fit in a seemingly fruitless fitness routine, Francine turned to yo-yo dieting.

After years of unhappily yo-yoing, Francine ran into an old friend who was stuck in a similar weighty predicament. They decided to be running partners, in hopes of reclaiming their pre-30s shape. In order to reap great rewards, they knew they needed to aim high—a marathon. Training was intense. It forced Francine to look inward and up her perceived threshold for pain and exhaustion. Each morning she would get up at 5 A.M. to run before what often turned into 14-hour days at work. As an advertising creative director, Francine did not control her own life, work did. Unfortunately, office hours often rolled into drinks, followed by dinners with clients. The only time that she had to herself was in the morning. With running shoes strapped to her feet and upward of 50 miles logged per week, dawn was her time to create some semblance of balance and serenity. After the marathon, Francine suffered from knee and hip pain, preventing her from sustaining her workout regimen at the same intensity. Simultaneously, she began to suffer from severe stomachaches caused by lactose intolerance—the inability to properly digest dairy. To correct the problem, her doctors recommended that she completely cut all dairy and most carbohydrates from her diet. She was forced to establish new eating habits, loading up on lean meats and vegetables. Sure enough, any excess weight began to fall off, but, without an exercise program, she lacked an emotional outlet to help diffuse her high-stress state.

One Saturday afternoon, Francine strolled into the office (a regular Saturday occurrence), and ran into a colleague who was oddly limping around the hallways. Expressing concern for her seemingly injured office mate, Francine asked what had happened. The response? Cardio Barre! A girlfriend had dragged her into a Cardio Barre class that morning and her body was already sore! Francine's immediate thought was, I want that. It had been a long time since she felt that good-pain burn that only intense exercise can generate. The limping is only an unfortunate side effect. A few days later, Francine stepped foot into her first Cardio Barre class. Though generally outgoing in a group, this class embodied Francine's cry for help. It was the admission that she had allowed an element of herself to spin out of control, and this class was her attempt to recapture her fleeting spirit. Sometimes, looking inside can be the hardest thing to do. She held on to the barre and thought, "Okay I am now embarking on something new." As a little girl, Francine took ballet classes, an experience that she thought she could draw upon to give her a leg up in class. It didn't. She was surprised to find that she did not feel flexible or strong. In fact, despite the fact that she considered herself a proficient runner with well-developed endurance, she was shocked by how challenging she found the class to be. Even her legs, which for years had been her predominant power source, quivered during many of the exercises. But, regardless of the musculature fatigue that she felt, her bones and joints were pain-free. That was it, she was addicted!

The next day, just as what happened to her office mate, she had a hard time walking. Muscles that she didn't even know existed ached. After years of running and aerobics, this class was changing the way in which her body moved and how her energy was dispersed. Unlike other classes, Cardio Barre forces you to be in control of your body. It is not about explosive, injury encouraging, movements. Your body is not propelled to move through speed or spring. Muscles are forced to work harder as you exercise control. It is both physically and mentally challenging. It is like a therapy session, intense cardio workout, and resistance training wrapped into one.

Francine came to depend on class for strength and energy. A self-described overachiever with a type-A personality, Cardio Barre became her essential outlet for momentary reprieve from life's stresses. She was filled with more energy and clarity of thought. She slept better each night, making her more effective and efficient at work. More than providing mental relief, her body began to change. Within the first month she noticed that she had became more flexible and her abdominal area (her "problem" area) started tightening. Even at her thinnest she had always had a little belly, but that was finally changing. Her arms became stronger and she shed the bra-strap fat on her back. Even her posture dramatically improved, warranting a slew of compliments on a daily basis. Of course, all of the positives compounded and fed her self-esteem, which is now higher and healthier. If you want to know numbers, Francine has lost 25 pounds and dropped to a size 4! For Francine, Cardio Barre is more than just a workout; it has changed her life.

15

Cardio Living

You don't need to dedicate yourself to a full-fledged exercise class every time you work out. It is easy to interweave exercise into your daily activities. Think about it, how many waking hours do you spend each day sitting, standing in line, leaning against a counter, or lying down? Let me lay it out for you room by room.

You can add a few minutes or even a few seconds of effective exercise while you are:

Kitchen
- washing dishes
- stir-frying vegetables
- emptying the dishwasher
- mindlessly looking into the refrigerator
- stirring, mixing, or folding ingredients

Laundry Room
- hand-washing clothes
- loading the washing machine
- folding laundry
- ironing

Bedroom
- lying in bed before getting up
- lying in bed before falling asleep
- deciding what to wear
- reading

Bathroom
- brushing your teeth
- taking a shower
- washing your face
- putting on makeup

Living Room
- watching TV
- talking on the phone
- vacuuming
- mopping
- sweeping

Office
- checking your email
- talking on the phone
- writing

Out and About
- driving
- standing in line

■ sitting in a movie theatre
■ at the dog park

How? You ask. It is easy. A few of the exercises are universal and can be done discretely without anyone ever noticing. Of course, some of the exercises are location-appropriate and I would advise that you use your own discretion as to when you should and should not try them.

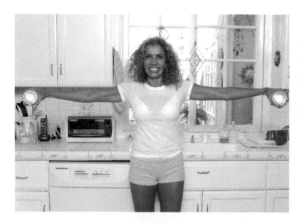

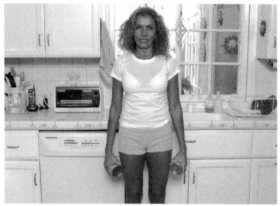

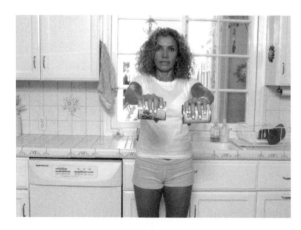

Kitchen

Pantry

FOOD WEIGHTS

- Tins of food, hand-size bottles or cans of soft drinks make excellent hand weights for arm exercises. Use them just as you might use a set of weights: Stand with your legs together. Hold the objects in your hands and allow your arms to drop at your sides. Slowly raise your arms out to your sides, up to shoulder height.

- Lower your arms down to your sides.

- Do 15 reps. Next, lift your straight arms in front of your torso to shoulder height.

- Lower down. Do 15 reps. These are great back and shoulder exercises.

Washing Dishes

HEEL RISES

■ Heel Rises are easy and discreet exercises that you can pretty much do anywhere: standing in line, talking on the phone, or when you are washing dishes. Stand straight with your feet together. Hold your hands lightly on the sink for support and balance. Lift your heels off the floor by pressing over the balls of your feet (but not onto the tips of your toes). Lower your heels back to the floor.

■ Do 15 reps. Heel Rises are great for your legs. Changing your feet position will target different sections of the calves. Turn your feet out and heels together to form a V shape with your feet.

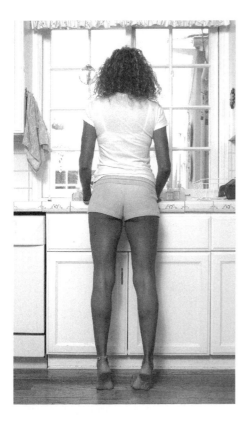 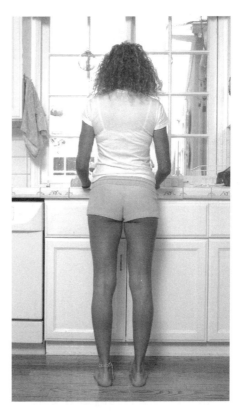

■ Repeat the Heel Rises in that turned out position for 15 reps. This will target your inner calves.

■ Turn your feet in so your toes are touching and your heels are apart.

■ Repeat the Heel Rises in this position for 15 reps. To target your outer calves.

COUNTER PUSH-UPS

■ Shape your arms with Counter Push-ups. Stand up straight a few feet from the counter. Face the counter. Place your hands on the counter to support your body weight. You should be angled toward the counter with your breastline at the height of the counter. Bend your elbows and lean your body into the counter. Keep the rest of your body straight—feet to head. Do not stick out your butt. Press away from the counter and return to your starting position.

■ Do 10 reps. Now you can wipe down the counter and load the dishwasher.

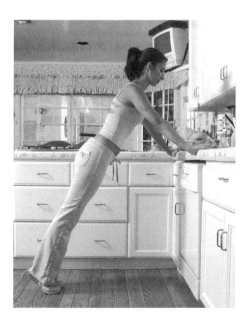
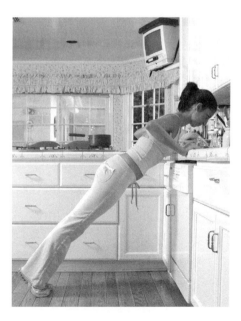

Mixing Bowl

CIRCULAR WRIST MOTIONS

■ When mixing batter or eggs, use Circular Wrist Motions to work your arms. Spend twice as much time mixing as you normally would (unless that excess mixing could sabotage your meal). Do not switch hands until your arm burns. Mixing a little longer is good for the wrists and forearms.

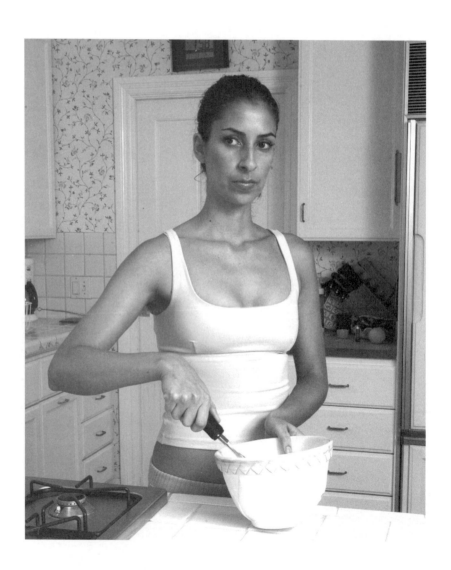

Boiling Water

COUNTER LEG RAISES

■ When you are waiting for the water to boil or the meat to broil, you can tone your legs with Counter Leg Raises.

FRONT LEG RAISE

■ Front Leg Raises will help strengthen and tone the front of the thighs while increasing hip flexibility. Stand upright with your feet together and your left side at the counter. Place your left hand on the counter. With your left supporting leg slightly bent, raise your right leg straight out in front of you up to a comfortable height. Keep your right leg straight and hold for 3 seconds. Lower it down to your starting position.

■ Do 6 reps and switch legs.

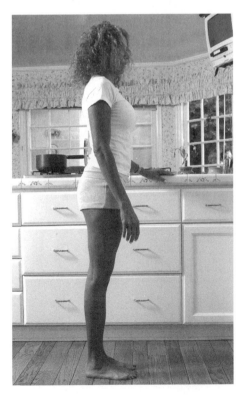 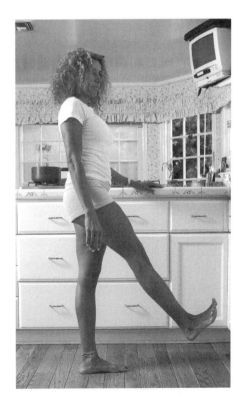

REAR LEG RAISE

■ To tone and strengthen the butt, lower back, back of the hips, and the hamstrings, do Rear Leg Raises. Stand up straight with your left side at the counter and your feet together. Place your left hand on the counter for balance. Lift your right leg behind you as high as is comfortable without bending your body forward. Hold it up for 3 seconds. Keep your buttock cheeks tensed throughout. It is harder, but much more effective. Lower your leg back down to the floor.

■ Repeat for 6 reps and switch legs. This is a slow and controlled movement. Do not rush.

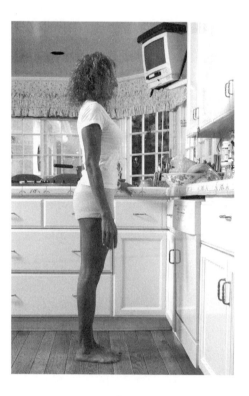
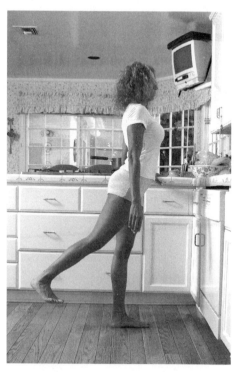

SIDE LEG RAISE

■ Don't forget to work out the sides of your thighs and hips. Side Leg Raises should give you that good healthy burn! Stand up straight with your left side at the counter and your feet together. Place your left hand on the counter for balance. Keep your body forward and hips straight. Your standing supportive left leg should be slightly bent in order to avoid locking your knees. Keep your toes facing forward to ensure that your hips stay even and straight. Raise your right leg out to your side as high as is comfortable. Hold your leg up for 3 seconds.

■ Return back to your starting position. Repeat 6 times and switch legs.

■ Increasing reps, holding for longer periods of time or adding ankle weights will make the exercises more challenging.

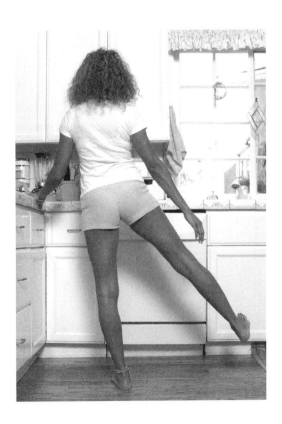

Laundry Room

Detergent Weights

SINGLE ARM BICEPS CURLS

■ Bottles of detergent have more uses than simply getting your clothes clean. Use the heavy bottle to do Single Arm Biceps Curls. Stand straight up with your legs together. Hold the detergent bottle in your right hand. Allow your arm to drop to your side so that the bottle is by your right thigh. Turn your palm so that it is facing forward. Bend your right elbow and curl the bottle up to your right shoulder, keeping your arm and elbow close to your body. Keep the movement slow.

■ Lower the bottle back down to your side. Do 10 curls and switch arms.

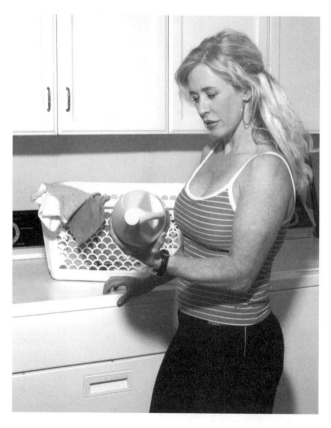

■ Strong biceps will help when pulling things and lifting heavy loads of laundry. Hand-washing clothing always takes more upper body strength and burns more calories than machine washing. If you have the time, wash your clothes by hand.

Ironing

IRON WORKS

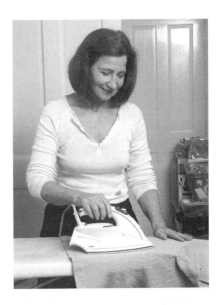

■ Weight Watchers translates 30 minutes of ironing into two points, which is the same as walking for 30 minutes. Iron once a week and do it for 45 minutes . . . this counts on the exercise charts! Also, walk in place while folding clothes.

WRIST SQUEEZES

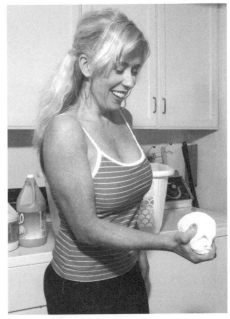

■ Roll up two pairs of socks into tight balls. Place one in each hand. Squeeze and release for a few seconds at a time. This will act like a stress ball and strengthen your grip.

ANKLE ROLLS

■ To increase ankle mobility and loosen your joints, stand with you hands lightly placed on the washing machine for balance. Lift your left foot a few inches off the floor and circle your ankle in a clockwise motion 10 times.

■ Reverse directions, circling in a counter clockwise motion 10 times. Repeat on the other leg.

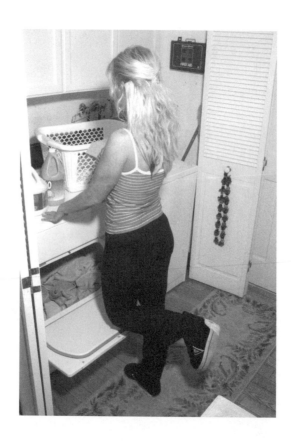

Bathroom

Brushing Your Teeth

THIGH SQUATS

■ Each morning and night you stand in front of the bathroom mirror for several minutes as you brush your teeth. Make use of those minutes and do some Thigh Squats to tone your upper legs and butt. Stand facing the mirror with your feet shoulder-width apart. Bend your knees and slowly lower your body down as if you were about to sit down. Keep your back straight and your knees directly over your feet. Slowly return to the standing position. You can do approximately 15 Thigh Squats during each brushing session!

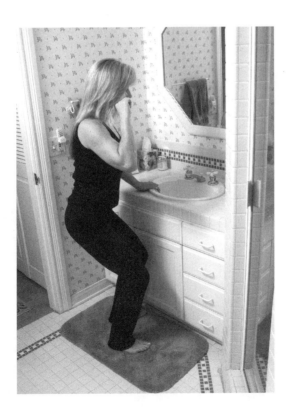

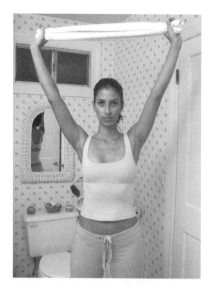

Drying Off
TOWEL STRETCHES

■ It is time to put your bath towel to more use! Stand up straight and place your hands on the lengthwise edges of your towel. Hold the towel above your head and pull on each end of the towel. As you pull, bend your torso side to side like a pendulum. Your head, torso, and arms should be moving in unison. Do not bend front or backward. This will improve posture, strengthen your core, and tighten your obliques.

■ Do 20 reps side to side.

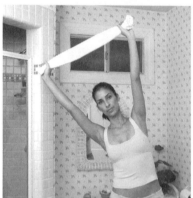

■ Lay a towel on the floor (it will stand in for a mat). Sit on the floor with your legs straight out in front of you. Hold another full-size

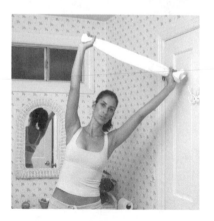

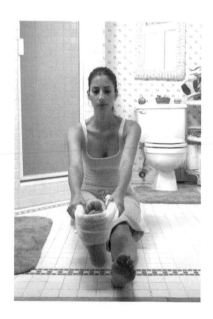

towel in your hands and loop it around the ball of your right foot (let your left leg relax). This creates resistance for your arms. Gently pull the towel with bothhands, stretching the balls of your feet back and lengthening your calves.

■ Repeat on the left foot.

■ While lying in the bath tub, raise one leg at a time above the water, hold for a few seconds and lower the leg down. Alternate legs. You can do 20 reps to strengthen your thighs and your abdominals.

Office

ACHILLES STRETCH

■ The Achilles Stretch is great for women who wear high heels because it helps to counteract the constant contraction of the calf caused by the height of the shoe. To do this stretch, slip off your high heels! Stand a few feet from a wall. Face it with your feet shoulder-width apart. Stretch out your arms straight and place the palms of your hands on the wall at shoulder height. Bend your knees as much as possible, but keep your heels on the floor. In this bent-knee position, breathe fully for 1 minute.

■ Repeat 5 times each day to stretch the Achilles tendon, which, particularly in females, shortens due to high heels.

■ While sitting at the computer, flex and point your feet to keep your ankles and feet strong.

INNER THIGH SQUEEZE

■ You might not think that a kick ball or basketball is appropriate at work. We are changing the rules! Place a kick ball or basketball under your desk where no one can see it. Sit at the edge of your chair and hold the ball between your knees. Squeeze your legs together, using the ball as resistance. Hold for a few seconds and release.

■ Do this 10 times.

HEAD AND NECK STRETCHES

■ We tend to hold a lot of stress in our necks. Avoid tension-induced headaches with simple stretches that can ease your nerves. Turn your head to the left so you are looking left. Hold for a few seconds. Return to central position looking forward. Turn to the right side. Hold for a few seconds. Return to center.

■ Repeat left and right 5 times.

■ Face forward and tilt your head to your left side so that your ear is closer to your left shoulder. Return to central position. Tilt your head to the right side. Return to center. Remember to keep a slow and gentle motion. No jerking. You will feel a gentle stretch on the sides of your neck.

■ Repeat 5 times.

TRICEPS PRESS

■ Sit upright on the edge of a chair with your legs comfortably bent in front of you and your feet flat on the floor. Place your hands beside your butt. Be sure that your hands feel stable enough to support your weight on the chair. Lift your butt and press up on the arms as your support. Your weight should be evenly distributed between your legs and your arms. Bend your arms, lowering your body slowly downward. Do not let your shoulders drop below your elbows. Push your arms back to a straight position, returning your butt to the height of the chair.

■ Do 10–15 reps. Make sure the chair is stable and is not on wheels. This exercise will quickly tone and tighten the flabby area on the back your arms (triceps).

Living Room

DANCE

■ If you have a small child, put on some music, dance around the room, holding your child in your arms.

ACTIVE TV WATCHING

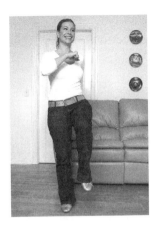

■ Walk, march in place, swing your arms around, lift weights, do tricep dips, leg extensions, or Pliés while watching your favorite television shows.

CUSHION SQUEEZE

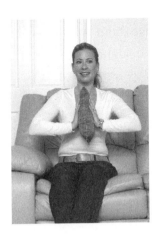

■ While sitting on the couch, hold your arms out in front of you. Slightly bend your elbows. Hold a cushion between your hands. Gently squeeze the cushion. Hold for a few seconds. Release. Breathe out as you squeeze and in as you release.

■ Do 6–10 reps.

DON'T FORGET YOUR FACE!

■ Just as you exercise your body to keep it tone, lean, and youthful, you can exercise your face. Ward off a face-lift by keeping your facial muscles in shape. Open your mouth wide, stick out your tongue, and move your mouth around in all directions.

■ Keep it up for 5 minutes. You can do this exercise anywhere, but be careful, it looks silly!

Cleaning House

CLIMBING STAIRS

■ To get your heart pumping and rev up your metabolism, try running up and down the stairs a few times. If your laundry is in the basement, take one load at a time and burn some extra calories.

SPEED CLEANING

■ Put on some fast-paced music and see how quickly you can clean the house. Speed-mopping and -sweeping not only get your floors clean, but they raise your heart rate, burn calories, and help firm up those sagging arms. You will also get the cleaning done faster and have more time for exercise.

VACUUMING

■ Use your upper back muscles by pushing the vacuum forward as far as you can and lunge forward with your right leg. Pull the vacuum back and return your feet together. Alternate legs. The heavier the vacuum, the more resistance it will provide. Move slowly to feel a good stretch through your back, arms, and legs.

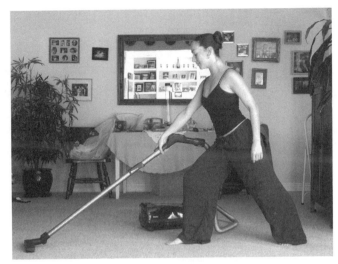

MOPPING

■ Fill two buckets, one with water and the other with cleaning fluid. Holding a bucket in each hand, slowly squat and lower the buckets to the floor, keeping your heels down and back straight. Keep your abdominals pulled in for strong back support. Stand and squat 10 times. Once your legs are pumped you are ready to clean the floor!

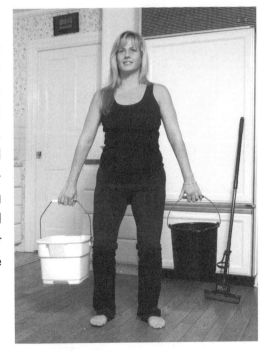

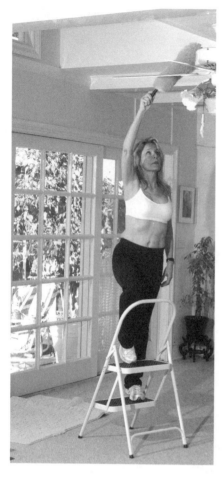

STEPLADDER THIGH BUSTER

■ Using a short stepladder, step up and down the ladder 10 times, alternating feet. While you are up there you can dust a shelf or two.

Driving

■ Whenever you go to the market, park your car at the far end of the parking lot and walk a little farther. The extra steps may not seem like much, but they add up!

■ Even washing your car can count as exercise. I mean really washing it . . . by hand. The car wash doesn't count! Wash your own car and burn extra calories.

GLUTE SQUEEZE

■ Whenever you come to a red light, squeeze your butt cheeks together and release to firm your butt. Do this for the duration of the red light to put that wasted time to good use!

Movie Theater

BALANCING ON LINE

■ While waiting on those long popcorn lines to get your food, slightly lift one foot off the floor and hold your balance for 10 seconds. Switch legs. No one will ever know that you are burning calories, improving your balance, and toning your legs. While you are at it, think about the healthier choices you are going to make once you get to the front of the line!

TUMMY TUCK

■ Tummy tucks (no, not the surgical kind) will help tone your lower stomach area. The best part about them is that they can be done almost anywhere, even in a movie theater! Sit upright with your back glued to the back of a chair. As you breathe out, suck your stomach in as tight as you can. Hold your stomach in, without taking a breath, for 3 seconds. Breathe in as you release your stomach. This simple yet effective exercise can also be done on line at the supermarket or lying in bed before you fall asleep.

Index